DIET JUST 2 DAYS A
WEEK AND DODGE
TYPE 2 DIABETES

2 Day Diabetes Diet

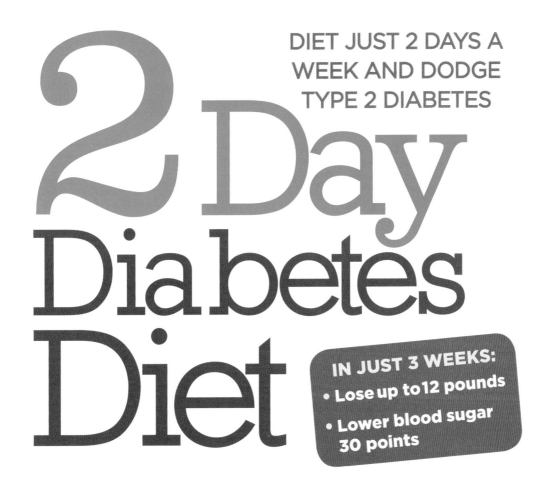

IN JUST 3 WEEKS:
- Lose up to 12 pounds
- Lower blood sugar 30 points

Erin Palinski-Wade, RD, CDE
with the editors of Reader's Digest
and Alisa Bowman

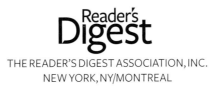

Reader's Digest

THE READER'S DIGEST ASSOCIATION, INC.
NEW YORK, NY/MONTREAL

A READER'S DIGEST BOOK

Copyright © 2013 The Reader's Digest Association, Inc.

All rights reserved. Unauthorized reproduction, in any manner, is prohibited.

Reader's Digest is a registered trademark of The Reader's Digest Association, Inc.

LIBRARY OF CONGRESS CATALOGING IN PUBLICATION DATA

Palinski-Wade, Erin.

 2-day diabetes diet : power burn just 2 days a week to drop the pounds / Erin Palinski.

   pages cm

Summary: "Based on groundbreaking new science, diet just 2 days a week to drop the pounds and dodge type 2 diabetes! In just 3 weeks lose up to 12 pounds and lower blood sugar 30 points! The plan is the culmination of the best research and studies from the world's leading universities and hospitals on the foods and eating strategies that help both people with diabetes and those at risk to lose weight and lower blood sugar. Based on the findings of a British medical study which showed the way to lowering insulin resistance by 22%, Reader's Digest worked with dietitian and certified personal trainer, Erin Palinski, to turn this research into an easy-to-use, easy-to-follow diet" Provided by publisher.

 Includes bibliographical references and index.

 ISBN 978-1-62145-104-4 (hardback) -- ISBN 978-1-62145-106-8 (epub)

 1. Diabetes--Diet therapy--Recipes. 2. Reducing diets--Recipes. I. Title. II. Title: Two day diabetes diet.

 RC662.P34 2013

 41.5'6314--dc23

                                        2013017470

We are committed to both the quality of our products and the service we provide to our customers. We value your comments, so please feel free to contact us.

   The Reader's Digest Association, Inc.
   Adult Trade Publishing
   44 South Broadway
   White Plains, NY 10601

For more Reader's Digest products and information, visit our website:
   www.rd.com (in the United States)
   www.readersdigest.ca (in Canada)

Printed in the United States
1 3 5 7 9 10 8 6 4 2

NOTE: Reader's Digest thanks Nipro Diagnostics for supplying the TRUEResult© glucose meters used by our test panelists.

Note to Our Readers:

Biochemical measurements, clinical guidelines, and treatments for diabetes differ in the U.S. and Canada. America uses the milligrams per deciliter (mg/dl) unit measurement system, whereas Canada, and most other countries, uses the International System of Units (SI). The SI measures all biochemical measurements, including glucose, cholesterol, and triglycerides, in millimoles per litre (mmol/l).

In America, a normal fasting glucose level of blood sugar (after you haven't eaten for at least 6 hours) should be 70 to 100 mg/dl. In Canada, the normal level should be 4.0 to 5.5 mmol/l. (Canadian measurements include decimal points, whereas US rates are rounded.) Canadians shouldn't be alarmed by the high figures for glucose targets used in America; instead, they must abide by Canadian guidelines.

To convert American glucose units to Canadian glucose units, divide by 18. For example, a glucose level of 106 mg/dl, divided by 18, translates to 5.8 mmol/l. To convert Canadian units of glucose to U.S., multiply by 18. For example, a glucose level of 6.5 mmol/l, becomes 117 mg/dl.

In terms of cholesterol targets, again there are differences between the two countries. Canadian guidelines urge people who are at moderate risk of heart problems to aim for an LDL level below 3.5 mmol/l and a total-cholesterol-to-HDL ratio below 5.0 mmol/l. In America, the guidelines recommend reducing LDL to less than 100 mg/dl (2.6 mmol/l) but do not set a target for the total-cholesterol-to-HDL ratio.

With cholesterol (which molecularly weighs more), the conversion rate to use is 38.67. To convert from American units (mg/dl), to Canadian (mmol/l), divide the American values by 38.67.

With triglycerides, a normal level in the US is below 150 mg/dl. In Canada, a normal level is considered to be 1.70 mmol/l.

If you have questions or concerns, or would like to find out more about diabetes, please contact the American Diabetes Association (www.diabetes.org) or Canadian Diabetes Association (www.diabetes.ca). Please note that the information in this book should not be substituted for, or used to alter, medical therapy without your doctor's advice. Please consult your physician for guidance before beginning this or any other meal plan.

Contents

What the 2 Day Diabetes Diet Can Do For You

In a breakthrough study, people who restricted carb and calorie intake just 2 days a week lost more weight and lowered insulin levels. We make this work for you in the real world.

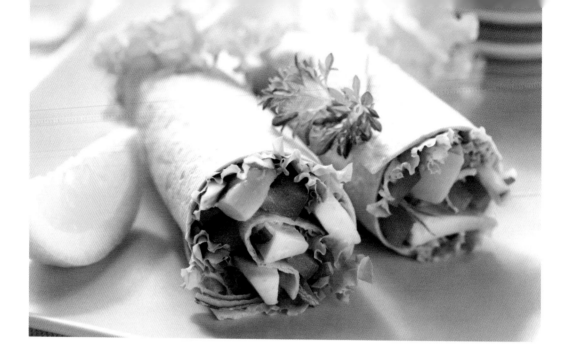

What will help you shed more stubborn fat and reverse blood sugar problems: shrinking portions 24/7 or dieting just 2 days a week? We're convinced that the answer will shock and delight you. That's right. It's the latter. *You can melt twice as much fat by dieting a third of the time.*

We almost didn't believe it either, but it's true.

When British scientists discovered this new 2 Day method for dropping pounds and normalizing blood sugar, it got our attention. So we enlisted Erin Palinski-Wade, a registered dietitian, certified diabetes educator, and certified personal trainer, to create an easy-to-follow program that synthesizes the research findings.

Then, to be absolutely sure of its effectiveness, we tested that plan on people just like you. They had diabetes, prediabetes, or were at high risk for developing blood sugar problems—and these problems had stacked the weight-loss cards against them. Their bodies seemed to cling to fat. Many of them had already tried a number of different diets and been frustrated by the results.

On the 2 Day Diabetes Diet, though, their results were startling. One panelist dropped 12 pounds in 3 weeks and 16 pounds in 6, more than halving her risk of developing diabetes![1] Another trimmed 6 inches from her waistline, while a third panelist dropped her fasting blood sugar by 30 percent over 6 weeks!

In a word: wow.

The World's Best-Kept Slimming Secret

You might be wondering: If this is so effective, why haven't I heard of the 2 Day method before? We'll tell you why. The researchers who discovered this new way of slimming down did not initially set out to create a new weight-loss diet at all. Rather, they were looking for strategies to lower women's risk of breast cancer. They knew that the consumption of fewer calories starves cells of fuel, which is actually a good thing in terms of overall health. Starved cells are less likely to divide and turn cancerous. For nearly 80 years scientists have starved yeast, worms, flies, and rats—cutting their calorie intake by more than half and consequently extending their lives by 35 to 65 percent. Various studies show that fasting—eating every other day, for instance—is good for us.

The problem: getting any reasonable human being with a healthy set of taste buds to not only try such a radical approach, but also to stick with it long term. Indeed, most people find it hard enough just to shrink their food portions a little bit. Could anyone realistically fast every other day for life?

Or was there a better way, one that allowed women to reap the cancer-preventing benefits of intermittent fasting without suffering from extreme hunger and cravings in the process?

As it turns out, there most definitely is. The researchers created a revolutionary new diet, one that was much stricter on 2 days of the week but allowed for larger portions the rest of the week. They then compared that approach to the typical diet that restricted calories 24/7.[2]

Their findings are as counterintuitive as they are exciting: Women who followed the calorie-restricted diet for 2 days a week but consumed larger portions the rest of the week lost almost twice as much body fat as dieters who restricted their eating all week long. They also reduced their insulin resistance by 22 percent. Additional work by other research teams has confirmed those findings and even suggests more health benefits, including protection of the brain against some of the effects of Alzheimer's and Parkinson's diseases.

A Diet That Seems like a Feast

For more than 90 years Reader's Digest has been discovering the most up-to-date, reliable, and useful health information and bringing it to readers like you who can put it to work in their lives. Our company library is full of health journals, and our team of editors and researchers scours them daily. You might say we're swimming in the latest health research. Even so, this study got our attention. Not only was it new, it was based on sound science. Scores of other studies—many of which you'll be hearing about throughout the pages of this book—supported the findings. Plus the diet itself seemed so doable. The first thing many of our editors thought when they heard about it was: "I want to go on a diet like that." We wanted to create a plan that took those stunning research findings and allowed everyday people with real lives—and especially people who have diabetes or are prone to developing it—to put them into practice.

So we asked Erin Palinski-Wade to create a simple and delicious plan to do just that. As a registered dietitian and certified diabetes educator, Erin has helped hundreds of clients in her private practice tackle blood sugar problems, the very problems that make dropping pounds so diffi-

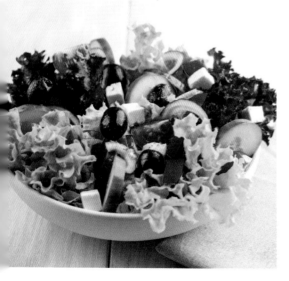

cult. Plus, as a certified personal trainer, she knows just how to tailor workouts to specifically help lower insulin levels. And as a busy professional herself, she understands that any eating and exercise plan needs to be flexible enough that you can follow it anywhere.

The result: the 2 Day Diabetes Diet.

You'll be happy to know that this revolutionary plan is not like any other diet you may have tried. You don't have to count carbs, calories, fat grams, or anything else. Nor do you have to banish the foods you love. Best of all: The special mix of foods and nutrients helps you fill up on fewer calories so you won't feel like you're dieting at all.

For this plan to work its magic, all you have to do is:

> **Power Burn 2 days a week.** Your low-calorie, low-carbohydrate Power Burn menu includes delicious soups, stir-fries, and satisfying homemade smoothies—all designed to satisfy your taste buds and appetite while whittling fat from your middle. Power Burn Days work at a cellular level to burn calories and reverse insulin resistance (a key factor in diabetes, prediabetes, and diabetes risk). You can choose any 2 days as your Power Burn Days; they can be spaced out during the week or scheduled back-to-back.

> **Nourish 5 days a week.** These menus include bigger portions, more variety, and a smorgasbord of soul-satisfying fare such as waffles, burgers, Healthy Chicken Parm (page 209), and Bean and Vegetable Tostadas (page 220). That doesn't mean you can pig out on these days, but you can enjoy reasonable portions of all your favorite foods. Trust us: You will not go hungry.

Power Burn Days work at a cellular level to burn calories and reverse insulin resistance.

Here's more: You'll eat 3 meals and 1 snack a day, even on your Power Burn Days. There's even room on this plan for chocolate, wine, beer, chips, cookies, and other decadent indulgences. You can still eat out, and exercise is optional (though recommended)! This is a delicious, family-friendly eating plan—one that you can keep up when you are busy, under stress, or traveling. There are modifications for people who are lactose intolerant or vegetarian, and we've even included several frozen dinner suggestions, too.

✻ What Our Panelists Are Saying about the 2 Day Diabetes Diet

How much did our first 2 Day Diabetes Diet testers like their new figures—and the new numbers on the bathroom scale? Here's what they have to say:

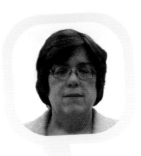

"I've had more success on this than any other weight-loss plan that I've tried in the past 10 years," says **Annette Sweeney,** age 55. She lost 14 ½ pounds as well as 6 inches from her waist and 4 ½ inches from her hips—even though her home lost power for days following Superstorm Sandy, which she notes "made cooking very difficult."

"I feel good," says **Karen Lerch,** age 52, who dropped 7 ½ pounds and lost 4 ½ inches from her waist and 3 ½ inches from her hips. At risk for diabetes, Karen also saw her fasting blood sugar drop 30 percent—from an above-normal 108 mg/dl (6 mmol/l) to a healthy 76 mg/dl (4.2 mmol/L). "(My) energy level is good and cravings are reduced."

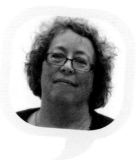

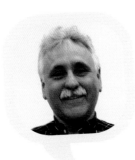

"I noticed results in just a few days," says **Ron DiLaurenzio,** age 61, who lost 8 ½ pounds and slimmed his midsection by 5 ½ inches and his hips by 1 ½ inches. "Positive changes were that I feel more energetic. I am better able to keep from snacking between meals and have less cravings for sweets."

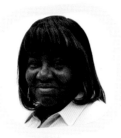

"On the second day, my morning blood glucose levels dropped," says **Edith Taylor,** age 57, who has type 2 diabetes. Her fasting blood sugar levels fell 40 points, from 192 mg/dl (10.7 mmol/l) to a healthier 152 mg/dl (8.4 mmol/l). That's a 21% decrease! At the same time, she notes, "My energy levels have increased."

"I started dropping weight pretty quickly," says **Jeanne Plekon,** age 60, who lost 16 pounds in 6 weeks. She also trimmed 1¾ inches from her waist and 3½ inches from her hips. "It works!"

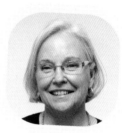

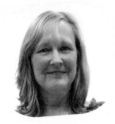

"I really like the recipes and the foods. My food cravings subsided," says **Nancy Taylor,** age 49, who lost 10 pounds as well as 3½ inches from her waist and 2 inches from her hips. "I was surprised by how tasty the food is and how easy the diet is. I noticed results within the first week!"

"The diet was so easy to adjust to, and I quickly lost my cravings," says **Mary Goudey,** age 58, who lost 4 pounds in 3 weeks and 6 pounds in 6. "I've finally found a plan that works and that I can follow for a long time."

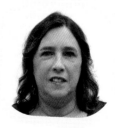

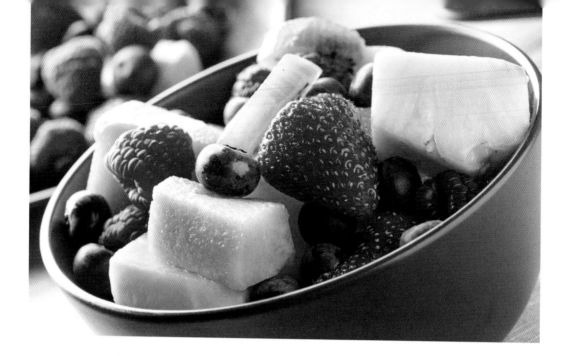

Lose Stubborn Pounds, Fat, and Inches—At Last!

We don't know about you, but we hate the idea of risking our health in the name of dropping pounds. That's why Erin went the extra culinary mile to make sure this plan boosts health as well as slims your body.

While most extreme low-carbohydrate diets skimp on fruit and even on some vegetables, Erin knew that the fiber, nutrients, and unique, hunger-stopping satisfaction provided by produce were way too important to skip. This plan's inclusion of fruits, vegetables, and even whole grains offers big benefits for your heart, your bones, and your brain.

But most important is this: This plan works. We tested it on a panel of 10 people, all of whom either had diabetes or were prone to developing it. The plan helped them take off weight, fling off belly flab, and trim inches. There was no waiting—weight loss started within days, several panelists told us. And several told us it was the most effective plan they'd tried.

What makes it so effective? Oh, the difference dieting only 2 days a week makes.

Drop pounds fast, even with a sluggish metabolism. The 2 Day Diabetes Diet is designed specifically for people with metabolism challenges. That's because it's harder for someone with blood sugar problems to drop pounds than it is for someone with a healthy metabolism. Blood sugar problems lead to metabolic changes that slow fat burning, and some of the medications used to treat blood sugar disorders can cause weight gain, too. On this plan you'll alternate between dieting days (called Power Burn Days) and nondieting days (called Nourishment Days). You'll Power Burn just 2 days a week, keeping calories and carbohydrates low. This, research shows, is precisely what people with diabetes need to heal their metabolisms and reverse blood sugar problems. On the other 5 days of the week, you'll nurture your metabolism with power foods that keep your body burning calories around the clock. If you add our muscle-building, fat-torching exercise routine and relaxation prescription, you'll reap even bigger benefits.

Thanks to the 2 Day method, you can achieve a healthier blood sugar reading within 6 weeks of starting the diet, just as our test panelists did.

Lose all the weight you want. You start a diet with high hopes, you lose a few pounds, and then, after a few weeks or months, you realize that you just can't keep it up. You adjust the diet as best you can, but the pounds start creeping back on. Soon you're back where you started. Sound familiar?

The problem is incredibly common. In a 2012 weight-loss study from Canada's University of Alberta, published in the *Canadian Journal of Surgery,* 43 percent of the program's 1,205 dieters dropped out before they'd lost a significant amount of weight—despite the fact that many had wanted to lose weight for years.[3] Why? Because their eating and exercise plans were too stringent, didn't taste or feel good, or simply didn't fit into a busy lifestyle.

On the 2 Day Diabetes Diet, you'll "diet" just 2 days a week—on the days of your choice. This ensures your success! If we asked you to follow a 600-calorie menu (or even a 1,200-calorie menu) 7 days a week, we're pretty sure your response would be two words: "fat" and "chance." But because we're only asking you to shift into high gear twice a week, the plan is doable. You'll be able to follow it long term—until you've reached your goal and beyond.

And keep the weight off for life. If you are a career dieter, then you know that dropping pounds is one thing. Keeping them off is another. In one 2012 study from the Wake Forest University School of Medicine, two-thirds of dieters ultimately regained their weight. On average, study volunteers had lost an impressive 25 pounds apiece, but put back 70 percent of it.[4] To prevent this frustrating yo-yo effect, the 2 Day Diabetes Diet teaches you a way of eating that you and your family can follow for life. Our test panelists reported that, after the initial adjustment period—

Are you ready to slim down and control blood sugar while you diet just 2 days a week?

which lasts a few days for most people—they found this diet so easy that they knew they could happily stay on it for the rest of their lives. And once you reach your goal weight, it gets even easier because you swap out Power Burn Days and switch to Nourishment eating 7 days a week. Our nutritionally balanced Nourishment plan will help you maintain your new shape for good. And if you gain a pound or two, simply add a Power Burn Day or two to your week until the weight is gone. Easy!

Are you looking forward to delicious, family-friendly (and easy!) meals like Grilled Chicken Kebobs (page 204) with pasta, Spinach Stuffed Meatloaf (page 199), and Round Steak Chili (page 180) with cheesy bread, and even Pita Pizzas (page 223)?

Tired of doing the "forever diet" cha-cha-cha—lose a few pounds, put your "big clothes" in storage, regain the weight, pull out the bigger outfits again? Wish it weren't so hard to lose weight with diabetes?

Are you ready to slim down and control blood sugar while you diet just 2 days a week?

The 2 Day Diabetes Diet is your solution. Dig in!

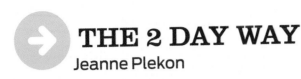

THE 2 DAY WAY
Jeanne Plekon

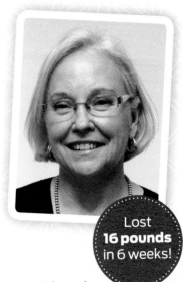

Lost 16 pounds in 6 weeks!

Jeanne Plekon, a 60-year-old IT director from Holmes, New York, had been diagnosed with prediabetes before starting the 2 Day Diabetes Diet, and she wanted to do everything possible to prevent herself from earning a full-blown diabetes status.

That's exactly what she did. She shaved off 16 pounds during her 6 weeks on the diet and even managed to stay on track despite being sick for part of that time.

"My goal on the diet was simply to lose," Jeanne says, "which I did—yay! But I had no idea what I would gain in terms of energy."

The key to the 2 Day Diet, Jeanne's way:

- ▶ **She did the cooking.** I wanted to follow the diet to a T," says Jeanne, whose husband had been the family chef. "So I figured, if I'm going to be a fascist about food, I should do the cooking. Because I typically get home from work pretty late, I did more cooking on the weekends, which meant I was thinking ahead and preparing early. That meant the food was taken care of, so I didn't have to sweat it on a daily basis. And my husband loved the food!"
- ▶ **She found a go-to meal.** "I discovered that the Subway just around the corner from where I work has a 6-inch, whole-wheat, all-veggie sandwich that meets the [guidelines]," Jeanne says.
- ▶ **She sneaked in dairy with an end-of-the-day shake.** "I generally had a hard time getting milk in my day, so every evening, I would do an end-of-the-day variation on the milk shake using 2 percent Greek yogurt, some unsweetened almond milk, and frozen blueberries," says Jeanne. "It was enough to keep me from feeling deprived."
- ▶ **She allowed herself one bite of a dinner companion's dessert.** "The first bite is always the best, anyway," says Jeanne. "After that, I can be smug. And that's satisfying, too.

CHAPTER **1**

Why You Need the 2 Day Diabetes Diet

Blood sugar issues slow your metabolism and make weight loss seem impossible. This diet tackles those issues head-on so you drop the pounds effortlessly.

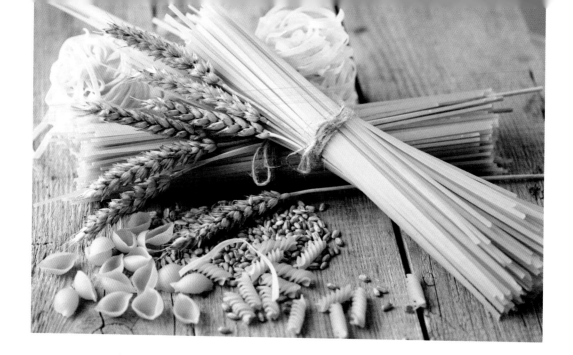

Maybe you picked up this book because you've just been diagnosed with type 2 diabetes or because your doctor tells you your numbers are moving in that direction. Or perhaps you don't have diabetes yet, but your family history makes you prone to it.

Whatever your reasons, know this: We designed this breakthrough plan specifically for *you*. The 2 Day Diabetes Diet's eating, exercise, and relaxation programs are calibrated specifically for people who have blood sugar problems or are prone to developing them.

That's important because blood sugar problems and excess body fat cling to one another much like dryer sheets cling to fleece. Perhaps you've noticed this already. Your doctor tells you to drop a few pounds so you can gain control over your blood sugar. You do your best to comply. Yet everything seems to work against you. You're so hungry that you're dreaming about food, so fatigued that a short walk with the dog feels like too much, and you crave the high-fat, high-sugar foods you are diligently trying not to eat.

Worse, even if you overcome all of that and manage to stick to your eating and exercise plan, the scale doesn't budge as much as you think it should.

Maybe you've even beaten yourself up over it all. Perhaps you thought that, if only you put in more willpower and effort, you would have dropped those stubborn pounds and reversed those climbing blood sugar numbers already. In reality, however, the problem probably isn't your willpower. Rather, it's this: The vast majority of diet plans just don't work for people with diabetes. Metabolic changes associated with diabetes may intensify hunger and cravings, slow fat burning, and encourage fat storage.

For lasting success, people with blood sugar problems need a very specific eating, exercise, and relaxation plan—the very plan offered in the 2 Day Diabetes Diet.

The Science of Stubborn Fat

Why do you need such a specialized plan? Blame it on diabesity.

Diabesity is the leading cause of disease worldwide. One in two Americans age 65 plus already have it, and epidemiologists predict that one-third of younger Americans will eventually develop it.

Diabesity is where blood sugar problems (diabetes) and excess body fat (obesity) meet, but the term is misleading because you don't technically need to have full-blown diabetes or obesity to be considered diabese. Just a small amount of excess weight or a genetic tendency for metabolism problems can be all it takes to set off a cascade of health issues, including high blood cholesterol, high blood pressure, immune system problems, and hormonal imbalances.

This constellation of health problems is caused by a modern lifestyle that is out of sync with our genetic inheritance. Because our bodies evolved with alternating periods of feast and famine, many of us inherited several different "thrifty genes" that cause our bodies to conserve energy (hoard fat stores) when calories are scarce and swiftly store energy (plump out our fat cells even more) when times are plentiful. Hundreds of years ago, humans with a robust set of thrifty genes were much more likely to survive long droughts and famines and pass on their genes to the next generation. It's for this reason that certain races of people—African American, Latino, Native American, Asian American, Native Hawaiian, and Pacific Islander—are more prone to diabesity. These races more recently survived periods of feast and famine. As a result, their gene pools are saturated with thrifty genes.

Flash forward to modern times. Now our thrifty bodies are confronted with 24/7 plenty. Those of us who live in the developed world no longer must walk for miles for a few hundred calories. We can open the fridge or any cabinet in the kitchen and easily find a few thousand of them.

For much of humanity, famine has dropped out of our modern existence. Now, all we do is feast.

As a result, it's incredibly difficult to maintain a healthy weight, and, once we gain just a little bit, the first hints of diabesity set in, making the upward progression of the scale hard to stop.

Many people assume that weight and blood sugar issues are a result of eating too many of the wrong foods.

> **You can trace your problems with blood sugar back to your mother and father.**

While this is true, it's only part of the story. In reality, you can trace your problems with blood sugar back to the day your mother's egg merged with your father's sperm to create the brilliant and unique you. That egg and that sperm probably came infused with DNA—a code of instructions— that caused your metabolism to be "thrifty." If one of your parents developed diabetes after age 50, you have a 1 in 13 chance of developing the disease yourself.

If one parent developed the disease before age 50, your risk is 1 in 7.

Both parents before age 50? You're at 1 in 2.

Having siblings with diabetes also makes you at risk, as does having other extended family members with the disease.

Among your thrifty genetics, there are probably genes that make your body more susceptible to an immune response called chronic inflammation. Any number of small, repeated irritations—including stress, poor food choices, and cigarette smoke—can trigger inflammation.

Here's what happens in the case of excess fat, especially excess abdominal fat. Fat tissue is rich in immune cells called *cytokines,* and these cells treat excess body fat like an infection. Although it's not completely understood why, one theory is that weight gain causes fat cells to expand beyond their capacity to support themselves, eventually causing these cells to die. This triggers cytokines to attempt to repair them. Once triggered, cytokines stand at high alert, ready to take down invaders like viruses and bacteria. The problem: The invaders aren't really there, but the cytokines don't cool down. Instead they behave as if they are fighting off an infection, and this leads to a host of problems. Although researchers aren't clear on the hows and whys, these high-alert cytokines activate several proteins that seem to dull your body's sensitivity to several key hormones, some of which may sound familiar to you:

Insulin: When you eat, the carbohydrates from your food are converted into glucose (or sugar) and are then absorbed into your bloodstream. Rises in blood sugar trigger your pancreas to secrete insulin. Insulin is a hormone that tells cells throughout your body to soak up blood sugar and either burn it now or store it for later.

When inflammation dulls your body's sensitivity to insulin, it renders your cells *insulin resistant.* That means cells don't readily soak up blood sugar when insulin asks. So your pancreas must pump out extra insulin to force blood sugar into cells.

Overly high insulin levels tend to cause dramatic swings in blood sugar levels, triggering hunger and cravings and causing you to reach for the very foods—fatty, sugary treats—that you've been trying not to eat. As you can probably see, body fat leads to inflammation, which leads to blood sugar problems. Blood sugar problems lead to cravings, hunger, and fatigue—all of which leads to more weight gain, which leads to more inflammation.

You can see where this is going.

Cortisol: This stress hormone is produced by the adrenal glands, and it's one of the hormones that helps us stay alert when, as one example, we are maneuvering a car through dicey traffic. Part of the fight-or-flight response, cortisol mobilizes our bodies for physical and mental effort. Among other things, it floods the bloodstream with glucose to be burned by the muscles for running and fighting. When cortisol rises and then falls back to normal levels, there's no problem. Problems set in, however, when cortisol levels remain elevated, which can happen as a result of chronic stress or chronic inflammation (or both). Chronically high cortisol levels hamper the effectiveness of insulin as well as keep blood sugar levels high. Because sugar stays in the bloodstream, it doesn't get to the cells that need it. Cells throughout your body then starve, triggering the release of several hunger hormones that travel to the brain, which in turn sends out its own set of messages that lead to hunger, cravings, overeating, and eventually, more weight gain. Once you've gained more weight, the cycle continues. Inflammation is now even worse, leading to higher cortisol levels and more insulin resistance.

Leptin: Secreted by fat cells, this hormone is supposed to travel to the brain and flip off your appetite switch. Think of leptin as being a caloric bank statement. It tells the brain, "Calorie stores are plenty." If not enough leptin reaches the brain, cells in the brain assume that calorie levels are low, and the brain turns up the dial on your appetite.

Excess inflammation, however, inhibits the effectiveness of leptin, preventing the hormone from completing its journey. Even though leptin levels in the bloodstream are high, not enough leptin gets to the brain. This is called *leptin resistance.* When brain cells don't receive leptin's message, appetite levels remain unchecked, leading to more weight gain, inflammation, and insulin resistance.

Ghrelin: Produced by the stomach, levels of this hormone rise when you've gone too long between meals. Ghrelin tells the brain, "The stomach is empty. Please fill it." The brain responds by intensifying hunger. As you eat, ghrelin levels fall, telling the brain, "That's enough." Then hun-

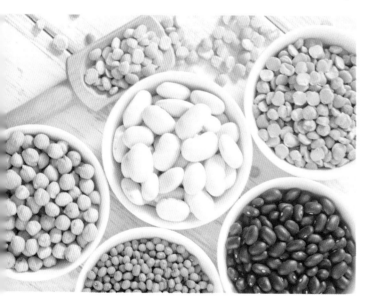

ger ceases. Inflammation seems to trigger an overproduction of ghrelin. This not only causes chronic hunger, it seems to encourage fat to be stored in the abdomen, which then leads to more inflammation and insulin resistance.

Even in the earliest stages of diabesity, levels of all of these important hormones are thrown off, worsening your struggles with blood sugar and body weight. And, as you can probably see, all of these problems worsen one another, creating a vicious cycle.

TURN DOWN THE THERMOSTAT ON INFLAMMATION

The 2 Day Diabetes Diet helps cool the systemic inflammation that leads to insulin resistance, body fat accumulation, and hormonal imbalances in several ways, but many other approaches worsen it. Here's how the 2 Day Diabetes Diet cools inflammation while other weight-loss plans and common eating styles fan its flames.

INFLAMMATION TRIGGERS (OTHER APPROACHES)	INFLAMMATION COOLERS (THE 2 DAY DIABETES DIET)
Foods with trans fatty acids (foods in the typical American diet, such as fried foods and processed foods)	Foods with omega-3 fatty acids and arginine, such as the fish and nuts showcased on your Nourishment Days
Foods with saturated fatty acids (such as fatty animal products), which are popular on unlimited low-carb diets	Low-cholesterol foods, such as the abundance of fruits, vegetables, legumes, and whole grains on your Nourishment Days
Blood sugar–spiking foods (especially the refined packaged foods popular in low-fat diets)	Blood sugar–balancing foods, such as the vegetables, fruits, legumes, and other fiber-packed foods on the 2 Day Diabetes Diet
Excessive exercise, like the type suggested in boot camp–style programs	Moderate amounts of exercise, exactly like those suggested in our optional exercise plan

So it's no wonder that ". . . in people with diabetes, weight loss may be more difficult than in people without diabetes," according to a 2007 weight-loss review in the journal *Diabetes Spectrum*. One of the first studies to document the struggle faced by people with blood sugar problems was published back in 1987 in the journal *Diabetes Care*. The scientists from the University of Pittsburgh School of Medicine put 12 overweight people with diabetes and their nondiabetic spouses on the same diet. By Week 5, the spouses were losing more weight. By Week 20, when the program ended, people with diabetes had lost an average of just over 16 pounds—impressive, but they were frustrated to find that their mates had shed nearly twice as much! [1]

This is precisely why you need a special diet. The 2 Day Diabetes Diet specifically addresses the metabolic issues that lead to diabesity, taking aim at all of the metabolic issues caused by blood sugar problems and excess fat—helping you to heal your metabolism and, finally, drop those stubborn pounds.

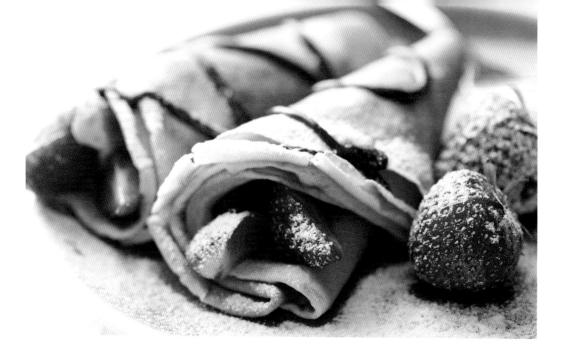

Diabetes 101

You don't need to have full-blown diabetes to benefit from the 2 Day Diabetes Diet. That's because the metabolic problems that lead to diabetes can simmer—nearly invisibly—for decades as your body struggles to keep blood sugar levels within a normal range. To understand how the 2 Day Diabetes Diet turns blood sugar and weight problems around, it's important to get a sense of how diabetes develops. Rather than think of the disease in black-and-white terms—that people either have diabetes or don't have it—think of it as the following continuum that starts with a tendency toward developing the disease and eventually ends with the disease itself:

Diabetes proneness: If diabetes runs in your family, it's likely that you inherited several thrifty genes. As a result, your metabolism is more fragile than that of someone who didn't inherit these genes. You're more susceptible to the effects of stress, poor diet, and other bad lifestyle habits, and more likely to suffer from inflammation as a result.

Insulin resistance: As mentioned earlier, your cells don't respond to insulin as they should. If you have insulin resistance, it's likely that other hormones—cortisol, ghrelin, leptin—are also affected.

Metabolic syndrome. Sometimes referred to as "syndrome X" as well as "diabesity," this is the cluster of health problems that result from inflammation and insulin resistance. You may have metabolic syndrome if you have three or more of these signs: a wide waistline, high blood pressure (even slightly elevated numbers boost risk), low levels of "good" HDL cholesterol, high triglycerides (fat in the bloodstream), or even slightly elevated blood sugar. This silent condition increases your risk of heart disease by 50 percent and stroke by 76 percent[2], as well as your risk for many types of cancer.

FAQ: WILL THIS DIET HELP ME IF I HAVE TYPE 1 DIABETES?

Type 1 diabetes is an autoimmune disorder that typically sets in during childhood. It is not caused by insulin resistance, but rather by the immune system attacking cells on the pancreas, eventually damaging the organ's ability to produce the hormone insulin. The 2 Day Diabetes Diet cannot reverse type 1 diabetes or eliminate the need for insulin, but it may allow you to improve your blood sugar control, lessen your need for insulin, and help reduce the complications of your disease. Consult your physician before starting this diet since insulin dosages and other medications may need to be adjusted to prevent hypoglycemia, especially on Power Burn Days.

Prediabetes: Insulin resistance eventually leads to a condition called prediabetes or impaired glucose tolerance. You have prediabetes when your pancreas cannot produce enough insulin to drive blood sugar into cells. Instead, excess glucose floats around the bloodstream long after you've eaten. Your blood sugar isn't yet high enough to be in the official range for diabetes, but you are moving in that direction. You have prediabetes if your fasting blood glucose is between 100 and 125 mg/dl (6.1 to 6.9 mmol/l). One in three American adults has prediabetes—including half of all people over age 65. And more than 9 million Canadians live with diabetes or prediabetes.

Type 2 diabetes. Once your fasting blood sugar readings are above 126 mg/dl (7.0 mmol/l), you have type 2 diabetes. (In Canada, doctors may also make a diagnosis based on the results of an oral glucose tolerance test (OGTT). With this test, a person fasts and then is given a solution containing 75 g of carbohydrate. Your blood sugar is checked after fasting and then again 2 hours after consuming the drink. Your doctor may diagnose diabetes type 2 if your blood sugar is greater than 11.1 mmol/l). According to the Centers for Disease Control, diabetes rates have doubled during the past 15 years. Some experts predict that, at the current rate of increase, as many as one in three people will have type 2 diabetes by midcentury.

No matter where you are on the diabetes continuum, you need a special diet, one that targets the two main sources of your problems:

inflammation and hormonal imbalance. Without that diet, you risk frustration—trying your best to stick to a plan that is working against your metabolism. And that's exactly what many traditional approaches do. Let's take a closer look.

Why Most Plans Don't Work for People with Diabetes

You can absolutely turn your metabolism around, but only the right program will get you there. Unfortunately, many of the usual approaches used to treat diabesity just don't work that effectively for people who have diabetes or who are prone to developing it. Consider the following.

Medications. One or more medicines may absolutely be needed for you to keep your blood sugar under control, and many of them are quite effective at helping you manage the disease. Some work by stimulating the pancreas to produce more insulin. Others block stomach enzymes that break down carbohydrates, and still others stop the liver from dumping glucose into the bloodstream. But taking medicines without changing your diet is like tying rags around your leaky pipes, but doing nothing to neutralize the corrosive water that is eroding those pipes in the first place. Medications treat the symptoms and side effects of diabetes, but they don't stop the cause: the foods and lifestyle that are leading to chronic inflammation in the first place. Case in point: Hundreds of millions of dollars are spent each year on the development of new diabetes medicines. As a result, the classes of drugs approved to treat diabetes have tripled in the past decade, yet diabetes is still the leading cause of blindness and kidney failure. If drugs were all we needed to reverse this disease, diabetes would have been cured by now.

Many medicines also pose undesirable side effects, ranging from gastrointestinal (GI) upset to weight gain. That's right: Medications used to control

> If drugs were all we needed, diabetes would have been cured by now.

blood sugar—including insulin, sulfonylureas (Diabinese, Amaryl, Glucotrol), and meglitinides (Starlix, Prandin)—as well as drugs that treat other health issues common to people with diabetes, including beta-blockers for high blood pressure and some antidepressants, may cause weight gain! Since excess body fat worsens blood sugar problems, it makes sense to do everything you can to follow a diabetes-preventing diet, thus reducing your dependence on meds.

Carbohydrate counting. Carbohydrates are one of the three nutrients in food that contribute to a rise in postmeal blood glucose. When you count carbs, you try to hold your consumption of carbs to a set number of grams at any one time. This prevents too much glucose from flooding the blood system at once. As a result, not as much insulin is needed to shuttle that sugar into cells.

While carbohydrate counting can certainly work, it's a complex process that requires a team of experienced professionals. Few people do it accurately without the guidance of a registered dietitian. It also involves studying your food choices in much the same way a baseball fan studies batting averages. You

FAQ: DO I NEED A DIABETES SCREENING?

Your blood sugar numbers are not only an important indicator of your overall health, they are also an indicator of your success. We recommend you schedule an appointment with your doctor and undergo a diabetes screening if any of the following are true.

▶ You are older than age 45.

▶ You have diabetes but haven't been tested in more than 1 year.

▶ You are younger than age 45 but are overweight and have one or more of the following risk factors: physical inactivity, previous diagnosis of impaired fasting glucose or impaired glucose tolerance, family history of diabetes, high-risk ethnic group background (including Asian American, African American, Hispanic American, and Native American), gestational diabetes or history of having given birth to a child weighing more than 9 pounds, elevated blood pressure, elevated cholesterol levels, polycystic ovary syndrome, history of vascular disease.

We recommend you get screened now and again after about 6 weeks on the 2 Day Diabetes Diet to see how well it is working for you. There are many kinds of diabetes tests. One common one is a fasting blood sugar test. This measures the amount of sugar still left in your blood after an 8- to 12-hour fast. Fasting blood sugar levels below 100 mg/dl (5.5 mmol/l) are considered normal. A reading of 100 to 125 mg/dl (5.5 to 6 mmol/l) is a sign of prediabetes; 126 mg/dl (7.0 mmol/l) or higher indicates diabetes.

Another common test is the A1c test. This measures the amount of sugar attached to hemoglobin in your red blood cells over a period of 2 to 3 months. An A1c of 5.6 percent or lower is considered normal. You may have prediabetes if your A1c is 5.7 percent to 6.4 percent. You may have diabetes if your A1c level is 6.5 percent or higher. Levels can range as high as 15 percent if diabetes is very out of control.

can't plan a meal without pulling out a thick book (or firing up an app) and checking all the carb grams of every food you plan to use in a recipe. Carbohydrate counting also doesn't necessarily tackle the underlying problems of inflammation and excess body weight. You can be an expert carbohydrate counter and still consume too many calories—thus continually gaining weight. You can also count carbs and manage to consume an exceptionally unhealthy diet—one devoid of important nutrients needed to calm inflammation, balance hormones, and reverse insulin resistance.

We're not against carbohydrate counting. You don't need to stop if it's working for you. For best results, however, we encourage you to combine your carbohydrate counting with the 2 Day Diabetes Diet. In this way you'll fill your body with the nutrients it needs to stop inflammation and other problems that are leading to your blood sugar problems in the first place. Eventually, once you get used to the 2 Day Diabetes Diet, you might find that you no longer need or want to carb count.

Glycemic index diets. The glycemic index (GI) is a measure of how hundreds of different foods affect blood sugar. All foods on the index have a numbered rank and are compared to glucose, which has a rank of 100. A food with a rank of 25 boosts blood sugar only 25 percent as much as pure glucose, a food with a rank of 50 only 50 percent as much, and so on. (Some versions of the glycemic index compare foods to white bread, instead of glucose, but the same principle applies.) As you can see, the smaller the number, the less a food is thought to affect blood sugar levels. Foods high on the index tend to be digested and enter the bloodstream swiftly, whereas foods low on the index take longer to break down, entering the bloodstream more slowly and evenly.

FAQ: I CARB COUNT TO CONTROL MY BLOOD SUGAR AND/OR SO THAT I GET MY INSULIN DOSE RIGHT. CAN I USE THIS DIET WITH CARB COUNTING?

If you don't already carb count for a specific reason, there's no reason to start. If you do, however, there's no reason to stop. Just carb count using the 2 Day Diabetes Diet's suggested foods, menus, and recipes as your guide. On Power Burn Days, you will have a smaller amount of carbs per meal than on Nourishment Days, so you would adjust your medication based on this lower carb level. You can carb count by using the Nutrition Facts panel on the foods you will be eating, the nutrition info or 2 Day Diabetes Diet exchanges of the meals and recipes provided in this book, or the diabetes exchanges created by the American Diabetes Association and American Dietetic Association. All portion sizes and exchanges in this book are based on the ADA diabetes exchanges.

Anything ranking below 55 is thought to be a low-GI food. Anything above 70 is considered high.

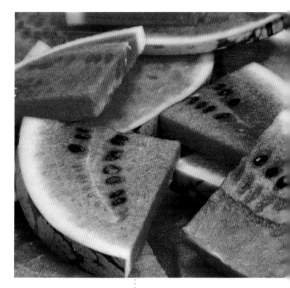

While the glycemic index is useful, it's not completely foolproof. That's because it's based on a fixed amount of carbohydrate (50 grams). But while you only need to eat one slice of white bread to consume 50 grams, for instance, you'd need to eat more than 6 cups of carrots to get 50 grams of carbs. Similarly, foods like watermelon (72), grapes (59), and bananas (62) score high on the glycemic index because they break down quickly, but actually affect blood sugar very little because they contain so little carbohydrate (because they are mostly composed of water).

A slightly different scale, called the glycemic load, is a bit more helpful, because it takes into account the actual carb content of a given food and the amount you would typically eat. A glycemic load of 20 or more is high, 11 to 19 is medium, and 10 and under is low. On this scale watermelon is a 4, grapes an 11, and banana a 16.

Still, while knowing the glycemic index and load of your foods is useful, it's not realistic to govern all of your eating choices by these numbers. With thousands of possible foods to choose from, eating by index or load can be even more cumbersome than carb counting. And when you combine foods—pairing a high-glycemic option with a low one—things get even more complicated. As with carb counting, you can manage to eat foods low on these scales that are devoid of the nutrients you need to heal your diabetes. For instance, white bread, at a score of 10, is low in glycemic load, but it doesn't provide much in the way of good nutrition. Shortbread cookies? Also a 10. And peanut M&Ms? They're a 6.

Low-carb diets. Similar to carb counting, low-carb diets drastically restrict your consumption of carbohydrates. This tends to blunt hunger, causing rapid weight loss. Here's the problem: These diets require you to nearly eliminate many foods that are actually quite good for your metabolism: fruits, starchy vegetables, legumes, whole grains, and dairy. They also encourage many foods that worsen inflammation, especially red meat. And they pose many side effects, including clouded thinking,

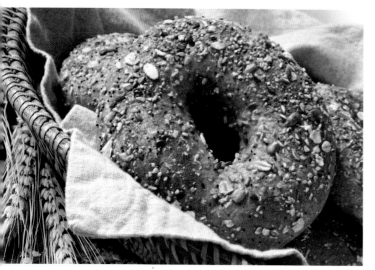

fatigue, and constipation. Perhaps most important, they are unsustainable. Studies show that many low-carb dieters cheat from the very beginning of these diets, consuming way more carbohydrates than the diets recommend. And the vast majority of people who drop pounds on low-carb diets generally gain those pounds back because they couldn't follow the diet for life.

On the 2 Day Diabetes Diet, you'll restrict carbs just 2 days a week rather than every single day. And even on your carb-restricted Power Burn Days, you'll be consuming nearly twice as many carbohydrates as you would on a strict low-carb diet. This allows you to consume the foods you love (especially fruit and grains), but still keep blood sugar low as well as drop pounds.

Extreme low-calorie diets. Some authors prescribe extremely restrictive plans that are simply unsustainable over the long term—our willpower can only hold out so long. Such plans recommend you subsist on a small variety of foods—often shakes, soups, or bars—and very few calories, often only 800 a day. They usually result in rapid weight loss in the beginning. The problem: When we constantly starve ourselves, our bodies want to keep us alive, so our metabolic set point adjusts. In other words, our metabolism slows. End result: Our weight loss slows and eventually stalls despite how few calories we may be eating. On the 2 Day Diabetes Diet, you will go very low calorie 2 days a week, but eat a more robust 1,500 calories on your other days. This not only is more sustainable, it helps trick your body, preventing your metabolic set point from readjusting.

Minimeal diets. Some plans do the opposite of extreme diets, suggesting that we eat every 3 hours to keep our blood sugar levels up. Their intention is good—extreme blood sugar dips and spikes are generally not healthy, and we're right to want to avoid them. But it's really difficult to consume the right number of calories six times a day. If you've ever tried it, then you know about this firsthand. Sure, your blood sugar never dips, but neither does the scale. It's okay to split up your meals throughout the day if you need to do so to prevent low blood sugar. Just be very careful to make sure you are consuming the right portions and right number of calories (as you will on this plan). Don't rely on minimeals alone to control your weight.

Portion control. Calorie counting can help you lose weight, but much like carb counting, it doesn't necessarily help you heal your metabolism, especially if you reign in calories while still eating a lot of junk food.

Hard-core exercise. Many hard-core fitness programs are hitting the market these days. They require lots of jumping rope and other strenuous calisthenics. While exercise is generally a good way to improve insulin sensitivity, intense exercise isn't the best way to get started, especially for people with diabetes or who are prone to it. For one, diabetes puts you at a higher risk for blood vessel damage in your eyes, and intense calisthenics can worsen that risk. Two, blood sugar problems tend to result in fatigue, a problem that makes exercise—especially intense exercise—quite difficult.

Also, exercise alone usually isn't enough to result in lasting weight loss. If it were, the phrase "overweight marathoner" would be an oxymoron. But it's not. Plenty of long-distance runners are overweight, and it's because they are not watching what they eat. On the other hand, you can drop pounds by dieting alone.

It's for all of those reasons and more that our exercise plan is both moderate and optional.

> The diet is specifically designed to cater to our thrifty genes.

What Does Work?

You guessed it: the 2 Day Diabetes Diet. While many nutritional plans work against your unique needs, the 2 Day Diabetes Diet works with you. In fact, it is specifically designed to cater to those thrifty genes that set you up for these problems in the first place. The 2 Day Diabetes Diet reverses diabesity primarily with something called modified, intermittent fasting. Don't worry, it's not as scary as it might sound. Here's what it entails. On Power Burn Days, you'll put weight loss in high gear by consuming about 600 to 650 calories. That's probably less than half what you are currently eating, and research shows that it's precisely this form of modified fasting that helps to reverse inflammation and normalize the function of insulin, leptin, and cortisol. By dramatically reducing your calorie and carbohydrate consumption 2 days a week, the 2 Day Diabetes Diet tricks your metabolism into thinking that it is living in the very feast or famine times for which it has evolved. There's lots of science to back this up, and you'll be able to read all about it in Chapter 3.

When you are not power burning on the 2 Day Diet, you are nourishing. Five days a week you'll fill your plate with foods from the Mediterranean that are proven to cool inflammation and reverse insulin resistance. We've minimized inflammation-producing red meat, sweets, and other processed and packaged foods packed with unhealthy fats and refined carbohydrates. Instead, the focus is on nourishing foods like produce, low-fat dairy, and good fats that flood your body with important vitamins, minerals, antioxidants, fiber, and fatty acids that cool inflammation, heal hormonal imbalances, control blood sugar and cholesterol, and even quell hunger pangs.

If you choose, you can then boost your results even further by incorporating our optional Tension Taming plan. This simple and quick relaxation program will help drive down cortisol levels, making both blood sugar and body weight easier to control. You'll find a number of Tension Tamers to choose from in Chapter 10, and we encourage you to try them on your Power Burn Days (or any day you need them!).

Finally, as we've mentioned, it's not always easy to exercise at the start of a diet, especially when blood sugar is out of control. That said, exercise is important. It helps build and maintain the muscle your body needs to sop up blood sugar. Exercise also helps make cells throughout your body more insulin sensitive.

That's why we highly recommend it. On the 2 Day Diabetes Diet, you can start your exercise program now if you feel ready, or you can wait until later. Either way, you'll find a realistic set of exercise suggestions in Chapter 11. Our walking and strength-training plans are tailor made for people with diabetes. They will help you turn around those blood sugar readings without causing extreme fatigue in the process.

One Pound of Prevention at a Time

Research shows that weight loss is one of the most effective ways to stop and reverse diabetes, and many of our test panelists experienced swift and dramatic results on the 2 Day Diabetes Diet. As we've mentioned, one dieter lost more than 12 pounds in just 3 weeks.

That's a lot of weight, but try not to get fixated on those numbers. Yes, you might experience similar success, and we are certainly rooting for you! But aiming for high weight-loss numbers is one of the biggest downfalls of most dieters. While you might be the breed of superhuman who can live up to these kinds of expectations, research has repeatedly shown that all-or-nothing approaches to weight loss typically end up doing just that—nothing.[3] A study published in the *Journal of the American Dietetic Association* found that half of overweight and obese study participants had unrealistic goals—especially the younger folks—and they expected to lose about twice as much as their doctors were recommending.

On average, our dieters lost nearly 7 pounds in 3 weeks and 9 pounds in 6, or between 1 and 2 pounds a week. That's a realistic goal, and it's one that can dramatically turn your diabetes around. Losing just 2 pounds drops your diabetes risk by a whopping 16 percent, finds research published in the American Diabetes Association's journal *Diabetes Care*.[4] Shedding only 11 pounds lowers your risk by 55 percent.

In a different study by the Centers for Disease Control and Prevention, small amounts of weight loss added up to a big difference. People with BMIs over 35 had an 83 percent higher chance of premature death compared to normal-weight people. But for people who had a BMI between 30 and 34—who were still technically obese—the risk was only 20 percent higher. And the people who were in the "overweight" category, with BMIs between 25 and 29.5, had no greater risk than people of normal weight.[5] Your healthiest weight will ultimately be the weight at which you can eat regular meals and exercise without dramatic fluctuations in weight.

> **If you've tried and tried and tried to lose, stop the insanity!**

If you've tried and tried and tried to lose 20, 30, 50 pounds and always ended up back where you started, stop the insanity. Our advice on this one? Shoot low.

Start the 2 Day Diabetes Diet by telling yourself you'll lose 1 pound this week. That's it! All you have to lose is 1 pound.

Chances are, if you stick to this program, you'll lose at least that the first week, maybe several more—and won't that be a delightful surprise? Then, you can use that momentum to set your modest goals for the next week, and the next—and continue to blast past those goals. Sure, you might have an overall range of 20 or 30 pounds that you're aiming for, but you're much more likely to achieve your goals if you take baby steps—and then are totally blown away by your own success.

To find out how dieting for just 2 days a week will help you drop that first pound and then the next and the next until you reach your goal, turn the page and read on. That's what the next chapter is all about.

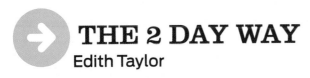

THE 2 DAY WAY
Edith Taylor

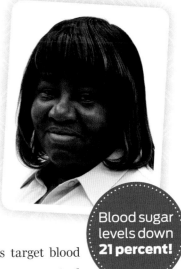

Blood sugar levels down 21 percent!

Sweepstakes promotional buyer Edith Taylor knows the equivalent of a winning lotto number when she receives it. And that's just what the 57-year-old got within a week of beginning the 2 Day Diabetes Diet. "I noticed a distinct change in my blood sugar level after just one Power Burn Day," says the Peekskill, New York, resident. "My blood sugar in the morning was always extremely high—say, around 250, which is nearly double the American Diabetes Association's target blood sugar level for diabetics. The day after my first Power Burn, it was 190. And one post–Power Burn morning, after being on the diet for a few weeks, it was 172! I couldn't believe my eyes when I saw the result! I had to take it twice."

Taylor has type 2 diabetes and is on medication for both her diabetes and high blood pressure. She was striving to drop both weight and blood sugar on the diet, and while her weight loss lagged (she lost a total of about 2½ pounds), her blood sugar levels improved dramatically. Her final blood sugar reading as part of the test panel was an impressive—and unprecedented for Edith—152 mg/dl (8.4 mmol/l). It was still high enough to keep a diabetes diagnosis stamped to her medical chart, but an impressive 21 percent lower than when she started the diet.

"Grandkids," quips Edith, who has seven, "watch out! I'll be able to hang with you this spring!"

Why the 2 Day worked for Edith, in her own words:

> ▶ **She expanded her diet.** "I tried foods on the diet that I'd never eaten before—like the hummus, which I found out I really like," says Edith. "And so I was able to replace my cravings for unhealthier snacks with foods that were healthier and just as satisfying."
>
> ▶ **She limited her portion sizes.** "When I first saw how much food I was supposed to restrict myself to while on the diet, I thought, 'I'm going to die here!' says Edith. "But it was enough. Actually, it wasn't just enough—it was more than enough, even on the Power Burn Days. I would never have believed it before I actually tried it, but some days, I had a hard time fitting in the snack."

Why You'll Love Dieting Just 2 Days a Week

Fasting primes your body to burn fat fast. We adapt this ancient practice into an incredibly powerful diet that's easy to follow.

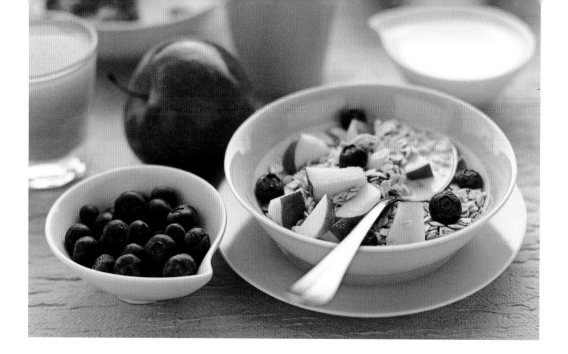

It's amazing—and true: Slashing calories just 2 days a week is a better way to prevent diabetes and lose weight than counting calories 7 days a week!

Why on earth would this 2 Day approach work? To understand the answer to that question, you need a little background.

For years researchers have known that severe calorie restriction can boost health. Just about every living being that researchers have studied—ranging from worms to fish to rats to dogs to monkeys—lives longer when it consumes one-third to one-half fewer calories. Calorie-restricted animals are less likely to develop diseases like diabetes, and humans who follow the eating approach have less inflammation, lower blood cholesterol, and lower blood pressure than people who don't.[1] People on severely calorie-restricted plans also have hearts that function like the hearts of people roughly 15 years younger, found one study.[2] Although scientists don't know precisely why severe calorie restriction works, they suspect it pushes the body into a type of cellular hibernation. All nonvital cell processes either slow down or stop altogether. This gives cells throughout the body more time to repair damaged components and patch up DNA. Cells and tissues age more slowly and turn off the problems that lead to cancer and poor health before those problems become unmanageable.

> **Every living being that researchers have studied lives longer when it consumes one-third to one-half fewer calories.**

Still, an old joke goes like this: Calorie restriction might help you live a decade longer, but your life will feel at least three decades longer.

Think of every plate of food you consume in a day. Mentally slash what's on it in half. Feel a little nervous just thinking about it? We're with you, and that's precisely why severe calorie restriction never caught on. Who wants to slash calories so severely? Not us, and probably not you, either. That's why severe 24/7 calorie restriction is not what we're suggesting you do for the 2 Day Diabetes Diet.

Because severe calorie restriction is so unpalatable for so many people, researchers have been trying to find a way to get the same benefits without the pain, hunger, and deprivation. For ideas, they turned somewhere you might find surprising: various world religions.

The Fast We Won't Make You Take

People have been fasting for religious and political reasons almost as long as there has been food on the planet. From studying these people, researchers know that our bodies finish absorbing and using all of the nutrients from our previous meal within roughly eight hours. Once that food is gone, the body then burns through stored energy in the liver and the muscles in the form of glycogen (a type of sugar). In roughly 12 to 15 hours, that energy is gone, too, so your fat cells start opening their doors and releasing their contents.

Hello, fat loss.

If a fast goes on for too long, however, things start to go awry. That's when our bodies start to sense that we're starving. Our brain turns down our metabolism, and our cells start burning a combination of fat and muscle protein. This isn't good. Muscle is metabolically active tissue that burns calories even when we're not using it. We need muscle protein to power our metabolism.

When they studied people who fasted for religious reasons—especially for the Muslim holiday Ramadan—researchers discovered, however, that the starvation cycle could be short-circuited. During the month of Ramadan, people do not eat during daylight hours. They only consume food before dawn and after dusk, so their bodies could be in a fasting state for up to 14 hours, depending on location and time of year. This seems to keep the body in a fat-burning state—the very state you want to be in when you are trying to drop pounds and reverse inflammation and blood sugar problems. Researchers from Qatar found that people who fasted for the holiday were able to boost the levels of the healthy HDL cholesterol by between 30 and 40 percent.[3] Other research found that this type of fasting reduced inflammation, blood pressure, and body weight.[4]

> Our ancestors lived this way: Kill bison, feast. Forage for berries, famine.

Of course, even Muslims only fast like this once a year for a reason. It's not easy to keep up. Still, given the health benefits of the approach, researchers wondered if there was a way to get the same results with much less pain and suffering. Enter the every-other-day eating approach. Eat one day. Fast the next. Then eat again. Then fast. Researchers reasoned that this eating style would mimic the lifestyle from which our bodies evolved. Remember that our ancestors lived this kind of lifestyle: Kill bison, feast. Forage for berries, famine. Early humans never knew when another unfortunate bison would stroll by, so when luck befell them, they ate until they were sated. The rest of the time our ancestors consumed only a light number of calories or, quite often, no calories at all.

Researchers soon learned that the theory had merit. When people ate every other day, they boosted health and peeled off the pounds.

But you know what? Intermittent fasting can make one's life feel even longer than severe calorie restriction does, don't you think?

Then came diets that suggested fasting every 3 days. Better, but still not tempting, right?

Thankfully, researchers at the Genesis Prevention Center at the University Hospital in South Manchester, England, came up with a much better way, one that achieves the same results but doesn't feel like a diet at all.

✳ What Our Panelists Are Saying about Power Burn Days

Wondering just how hard it is to make it through a Power Burn Day? Here's what some volunteers who tried the 2 Day Diabetes Diet had to say about it:

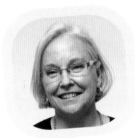

"I figured that on days where I'd be giving myself less fuel that I'd wake up the next day feeling sluggish. But I didn't—the mornings after Power Burn Days, I would wake up early. Trust me: The 2 days a week are not hard. And they work."

—**Jeanne Plekon**

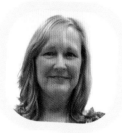

"The first few were tough, but I drank a lot of water to help me cope with any hunger."

—**Nancy Taylor**

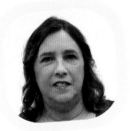

"On Power Burn Days I ate big cups of vegetable soup. This saved me."

—**Mary Goudey**

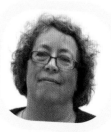

"I'm a soup girl, so I really like the broth. It's comforting to me, and I really enjoy it. So I'm not hungry on Power Burn Days—or on any days of the diet."

—**Karen Lerch**

The Birth of the 2 Day Diet

The 2 Day Diabetes Diet was inspired by a groundbreaking British study that has challenged and changed conventional wisdom about the best way to lose weight, trim inches, blast belly fat, and get healthier.[5] Rather than eat nothing at all during fasting days, these British researchers allowed study participants to consume about 600 calories 2 days a week. On these days the researchers were able to restrict calories just enough to make the body think it was fasting, but not so much that their diet became impossible to follow long term. On the rest of the days, study participants consumed a more robust 1,500 calories.

Within 6 months, the study participants:

- ▶ Reduced inflammation an average of 15 percent
- ▶ Reduced insulin an average of 25 percent
- ▶ Reduced leptin an average of 40 percent[6]

The researchers then fine-tuned the approach, experimenting with the best makeup of foods, distribution of calories, and more. Their goal: to create a diet that not only soothed inflammation, dropped levels of insulin and leptin, and helped dieters peel off the pounds, but also was possible to follow long term. Based on their groundbreaking research as well as other studies, this is what we now know about the following dieting approaches.

Powerful, but impossible to follow long term: severely slashing calories in half or eating only every other day.

Easy to stick to, but not very powerful: following a wholesome, 1,400- to 1,500-calorie Mediterranean diet 7 days a week.

Incredibly powerful and easy to stay on: Following a super-low-calorie, low-carb diet 2 days a week and a Mediterranean diet the rest of the days. Women who followed this dietary approach lost nearly twice as much weight as women who dieted all 7 days of the week. They also lost more body fat and kept more lean muscle mass (crucial for maintaining a lower, healthier weight)! And their waistlines were smaller. Two-day dieters lost an average of 2 inches around their middles, while full-time dieters lost less than 1½ inches.

The 2 Day Diabetes Diet takes that incredibly powerful British approach but modifies it to work for people with diabetes, real taste buds, and busy lifestyles. On the 2 Day Diabetes Diet, you'll follow the powerful and doable 2 plus 5 approach to achieve lasting blood sugar success.

Two days a week you'll slash calories and carbs, but you'll still consume foods known to be important in controlling inflammation, blood sugar, and more. Although these foods are low in calories, they are still high in satisfaction. Thanks to the help of high-volume soups, filling salads, and rich smoothies, you'll fill up, but you won't fill out.

On the other 5 days a week, you'll fill your plate with wholesome, anti-inflammatory foods from the Mediterranean. These foods are so delicious that you'll have a hard time believing that they are diet foods at all. Take a look at the following chart to get a sense of what you'll be eating on this mouthwatering and effective plan.

Look doable? Sound like a plan you can definitely stick to? We sure hope so. Now here's more: Intermittent dieting isn't the only secret behind your 2 Day Diet success. Turn to the next chapter to learn the 2 Day Diabetes Diet's five key practices that can help you tame blood sugar and drop pounds—for the last time.

	2 DAYS A WEEK: POWER BURN	5 DAYS A WEEK: NOURISH
Daily Calories:	600 to 650	about 1,500
Type of Eating:	Low carb	Mediterranean
SAMPLE MEAL:		
Breakfast	2-egg veggie omelet + yogurt	Banana toast + yogurt
Lunch	Carrot soup + fruit	Turkey and hummus wrap + salad
Dinner	Meat loaf + broccoli + milk	Garden soup + pork tenderloin + sweet potato + collards
Snack	Grapes	Sliced apple

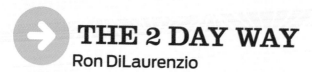

THE 2 DAY WAY
Ron DiLaurenzio

If computer programmer Ron DiLaurenzio could simply write a line of code that would ensure his protection from diabetes, he would do so—because his genetic code sure seems stacked against him. Ron's paternal grandmother had diabetes. His father and all his dad's siblings had diabetes. His sister has diabetes. His cousins have diabetes. Ron himself does not—"My blood sugar has tested high only one time," he says—and, having watched his dad go blind, lose two toes, and eventually die of complications from the disease, he aims to keep it that way . . . if he can survive the Power Burn Days.

"In general, I love the 2 Day plan," he says. "The good food choices made it really easy to create meals that I liked and that worked for me weight-loss-wise. But the Power Burn Days were really tough at first"—especially the day his car broke down and he had to walk 6 miles home because he had forgotten his cell phone!

The 61-year-old persevered by snacking on veggies to stave off his hunger pangs and by reveling in his almost immediate success. "I actually noticed results in just a few days," says Ron. "I felt—and still feel—more energetic. I crave sweets less. And I'm better able to keep from snacking in between meals." Ron lost 8 ½ pounds and an impressive 5 ¾ inches from his waist during the 6 weeks he was on the diet, despite allowing his nondieting son to move in with him during that period. "Having a nonparticipating person in the house makes for a lot of temptations," Ron laughs. "I wouldn't recommend it!"

The key to the 2 Day, Ron's way:

▸ **He followed the 2 Week Quick Start plan.** "The 2 Day Diabetes Diet was different for me because it was the first time I followed a menu," noted Ron. "That actually made it easier. I didn't have to count calories, since the menu was pre-calculated. Just cook it or mix it, and eat it! I think that helped a lot."

Beating the diabetes gene!

▶ **He split his meals in two.** "I was used to having a snack when I first got to work, since I usually eat breakfast by 5:30 a.m. To make it work better, I began splitting my breakfast in half and eating half at home, half at work."

▶ **He exercised!** Having observed that his father's decline accelerated once he retired and stopped being active, Ron has been doing some form of aerobic activity since his early twenties. "I was a runner for many years," he said. "I have always bicycled—doing a daily paper route for 4 years into my early teens—and have done century rides and other long rides or spin classes over the years. My father also did a paper route by bicycle when he was young (he actually rode much farther, and some of my customers had been on his route!), but he never did any regular exercise [like this.] . . . I found that I shed the weight a lot faster when I walk at least 20 minutes every day. Running, cycling, or doing other aerobic activities makes it go even quicker."

CHAPTER 3

The Five Practices of the 2 Day Diabetes Diet

Three required and two optional practices work together to cool inflammation, reverse insulin resistance, balance hormones, and help you peel off the pounds.

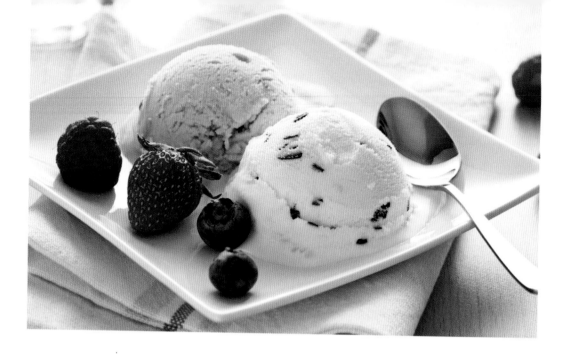

There's a lot to love about the 2 Day Diabetes Diet. For one, the plan is powerfully delicious. With goodies like dark chocolate and ice cream and hearty delights like Eggplant Lasagna (page 224) and Orange Beef with Broccoli (page 202), how can your taste buds (and your family members) not love this plan?

It's also powerfully inclusive. While other plans tell you about all the foods and food groups you can't eat, the 2 Day Diabetes Diet focuses instead on all the wonderfully metabolism-healing foods that you can consume. And, as it turns out, that includes a lot of foods. On this plan we not only allow you to consume dairy (including ice cream), we encourage it. Grains and fruit—both banned by low-carb diets—are back on the menu. And there's even room for alcohol and desserts. If you are a meat eater, you'll find plenty of stick-to-your-ribs options. If you are a vegetarian, we've also got you covered. If you're lactose intolerant, we've got plenty of options for you, too.

And it's powerfully flexible. Rather than hand you a set of menus and expect you to follow them regardless of your lifestyle, taste buds, and interests, we provide you with a three-level plan and help you choose the best level for you. We designed the 2 Day Diabetes Diet for real people with real lives. Each of our three levels is designed for different mind-sets and personalities. We're confident that you'll find a level that is just right for you.

▸ *If you are the kind of person who loves structure,* our Level 1 plan is a great place to start. Its detailed menus will walk you through the 2 Day Diabetes Diet. We've even compiled your shopping lists for you.

▸ *If you are the kind of person who enjoys some freedom,* the Mix and Match Plan in Level 2 will work great. It includes dozens of choices for every meal and snack. Whether you are a meat eater or a vegetarian, a slow-food convert or someone with an on-the-go lifestyle, you'll find the options you need for lasting success. We've even included grab-and-go, frozen dinner, and restaurant suggestions.

▸ *If you love to design your own recipes and meals,* our Free Range Plan in Level 3 will work great. It teaches you how to create your own Power Burn and Nourishment Days.

But what's most important about this plan is this: It works. The 2 Day Diabetes Diet includes five powerful practices—three required and two optional—designed to cool inflammation, reverse insulin resistance, balance hormones, and help you peel off the pounds.

Practice #1: Power Burn eating. When you eat to power burn twice a week, you hold yourself to about 600 to 650 calories—without hunger or cravings—thanks to three satisfying meals plus a snack. As you'll soon learn, this shifts your metabolism out of carb burning into fat burning. This not only allows you to finally shrink the size of those fat cells, it also turns down the demand on your metabolism and helps to put an end to inflammation and insulin resistance.

Practice #2: Nourishment eating. When you are not power burning, you are nourishing. On your 5 Nourishment Days, you'll increase the calorie count to about 1,500 as you enjoy Mediterranean-inspired meals featuring a bounty of fruit, vegetables, whole grains, good fats, lean protein, and reduced-fat dairy products. Your Nourishment Days are full of metabolism-healing foods that drive down inflammation, reverse insulin resistance, and balance hormones.

Practice #3: Satisfaction eating. We're sure there's a flavor or mouthfeel that you just can't do without. Maybe it's the crunchy saltiness

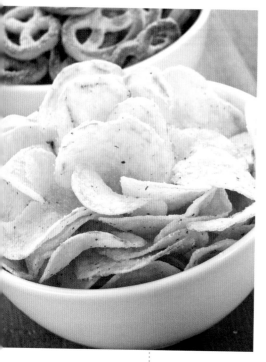

of snack chips, the creamy sweetness of chocolate, or the warmth of a glass of wine, beer, or liquor. Many plans make such treats off-limits, but this isn't so on the 2 Day Diabetes Diet. We not only allow decadence, we encourage it. Indulging twice a week will improve your success! By choosing from our list of nourishing treats, you'll not only satisfy your taste buds, you'll also help to drive down blood sugar, inflammation, and more.

Practice #4: Tension Taming. Stress not only leads to emotional eating, it also can boost inflammation and blood sugar, contributing to the vicious diabesity cycle we mentioned in Chapter 1. That's why we made sure to include an optional Tension Taming routine. You'll find it in Chapter 10, and we recommend you follow it at least twice a week, especially on your Power Burn Days.

Practice #5: Moving. Exercise is optional on the 2 Day Diabetes Diet. If you choose to do it, however, you'll banish cravings and hunger even more. Research shows that movement helps to improve leptin signaling, insulin sensitivity, and much more. You'll find an effective, easy-to-follow exercise plan in Chapter 11.

When you add up those practices, you end up with this: a powerfully effective plan that you can't help but love. You've already learned about the dangers of inflammation, insulin resistance, and hormonal imbalance. You've learned how the 2 plus 5 approach works. Now it's time to take a closer look at each of the 5 key practices of the 2 Day Diet, so you can learn how each piece of the plan takes aim at extra pounds, inflammation, belly fat, and insulin resistance.

Practice #1:
Power Burn Eating

Of all the practices we just described, the most unique, counterintuitive, and revolutionary, of course, is #1: Power Burn eating. There are two hallmarks of your Power Burn Days. They will be:

Low carbohydrate. On the 2 Day Diabetes Diet, your Power Burn Days include roughly 75 grams of carbs. That's less than half the carbs you're probably used to (the typical American consumes about 55 percent of their calories from carbs, which works out to almost 200 grams in a 1,500-calorie diet), but quite a bit more than the typical low-carb diet, which holds carbs to just 30 grams a day. That's both punishing and unnecessary. A more robust 75 grams of carbs is low enough to dramatically reduce blood sugar and insulin levels, but high enough to allow you to consume some of the foods you love. For instance, you'll still be able to consume two servings of fruit, two servings of dairy, and a half serving of grain on your Power Burn Days.

Low calorie. Power Burn Days are very low in calories, about 600 to 650 total. This is just enough calories to give you all the nutrients your body needs for health and well being. It's also just enough to be realistic, but still under your body's metabolic radar. Your cells will behave as if you are fasting, slowing down bodily processes so they can heal and come back stronger.

As we've said, the 2 Day Diabetes Diet is powerfully flexible, and Power Burn Days are no exception. You can power burn any 2 days of the week. If your life gets busy, you can skip a week or two of power burning and get back to it as needed. Generally, though, you'll use Power Burn Days until you drop all the weight you want and get your blood sugar under control. Then, if you'd like, you'll switch to nourishing 24/7, adding power burning back in as needed over time.

Your Power Burn Days may be low in calories and carbs, but they are high in satisfaction and effectiveness. Your 2 weekly Power Burn Days will help you to:

Lower blood sugar. Power Burn Days work by zeroing in on the very hormone people with diabetes most need to have under control: insulin.

Researchers at various institutions have consistently found that intermittent fasting primes cells throughout the body to absorb glucose more readily, making cells more insulin sensitive.[1,2] End result: Insulin levels drop. In the British study on which this plan is based, participants were able to drop insulin levels by 25 percent, compared to 4 percent for those on a full-time diet.

To understand why intermittent fasting makes cells more insulin sensitive, imagine a world without weekends . . . a world in which every Friday was followed by a Monday, with no break between. A pretty grim scenario, no? Whatever the demands of your job, family, or household, you probably wouldn't want to do without a weekly respite. Even if your schedule keeps you crazy busy on weekends, chances are you have some days of rest penciled into your calendar.

Turns out your metabolism—especially if you are carrying around a set of thrifty genes—feels the same way, and that's why Power Burn Days are so important to the 2 Day Diabetes Diet. Power Burn Days are like a weekend for your metabolism. It's the difference between a workday, when you have a million and one tasks clamoring for your attention, and a Saturday, when you can get the laundry done, plow through the bills that have piled up on the kitchen table, and generally clear the decks because there's time to breathe.

The lighter load of calories and carbs on Power Burn Days allows your system to rest. Because your body isn't overwhelmed with calories, blood sugar levels remain low. Because blood sugar levels stay low, so do levels of insulin. Because insulin levels stay low, your body can more easily access and burn body fat for fuel.[3]

Soothe inflammation. Giving your system this kind of periodic caloric and carbohydrate break does more than just lower insulin. It also enables your body to come back stronger and healthier. When you restrict calories 2 days a week, you switch your body out of growth mode and into repair mode. Your liver and other organs now have a chance to build molecules and repair damaged cells, preventing and reversing chronic inflammation.[4] In the British study, levels of inflammatory markers dropped 15 percent for women who dieted 2 days a week.

Normalize leptin. The British study uncovered something amazing about this 2 plus 5 approach: It lowers levels of the appetite-regulating hormone leptin by one-third to nearly one-half.[5] As we mentioned in Chapter 1, reduced leptin levels help to improve appetite signaling in the brain. End result: You feel less hungry. Lower leptin levels also lead to less inflammation and improved insulin sensitivity.

On the 2 Day Diabetes Diet, we help you to drive down leptin even more by keeping Power Burn Days low in sweeteners like sugar and high-fructose corn syrup. University of Florida researchers discovered in 2008 that fructose (from sweetened foods like candy and not from wholesome foods like fruit) tricks brain cells into ignoring leptin. In a lab study published in the journal *American Journal of Physiology: Regulatory, Integrative and Comparative Physiology,* fructose induced leptin resistance and triggered overeating. How does fructose fool neurons? The researchers noticed that high-fructose foods—like candy, soda, and baked goods, but not fruit—also boosted blood levels of triglycerides. They suspect the triglycerides then prevented leptin from reaching brain cells.[6]

Boost fat burning. During Power Burn Days, your body burns through all of its easily accessible sources of fuel such as blood sugar and fuel stored in the muscles and liver in the form of glycogen. Once it does so, it switches to fat burning. That's precisely what you want to happen when you are attempting to drop pounds.

Reduce hunger and cravings. We packed our Power Burn Days with exceptionally filling foods and beverages. These days are designed to be very low in carbohydrates and very high in both fiber and water-rich foods, all of which help to fill you up on many fewer calories. The combination of

FAQ: WHAT IF I FEEL LIGHT-HEADED ON POWER BURN DAYS?

Becoming light-headed can happen for a few reasons. Use the following advice.

Check your blood sugar. Light-headedness can be a sign of hypoglycemia, so take your blood sugar right away. See box on page 94 for more information.

Ease off on the movement. Exercise mostly on Nourishment Days and include only mild stretching and relaxation on Power Burn Days.

Drink up. Dehydration, even mild dehydration, can cause this feeling, so make sure to drink at least 64 ounces of water per day. (If you really need a change of pace, club soda, seltzer, decaf tea, and decaf coffee are also okay.)

Eat more often. On Power Burn Days, try spacing your meals out as six small meals rather than three larger meals, and avoid going longer than 3 or 4 hours without eating.

Replace sodium. Make sure you are including the recommended bouillon each day, since its sodium content can help to prevent electrolyte imbalances that can also cause light-headedness.

lean protein and fiber-and-water-rich vegetables helps in several ways. Protein triggers cells in the intestine to release just enough glucose to signal both the liver and brain to flip off your hunger switch. And fruits, vegetables, and other water-rich foods are heavy. They weigh down your stomach, trigging nearby nerves to communicate the "full" message to the brain.

Our test panelists confirmed this. Many told us that they didn't feel hungry at all. Others said they only noticed hunger initially, but they soon learned to snack on low-calorie foods like vegetables or to consume soup and even water more often (all strategies we promote on the plan). It didn't take long, they told us, before hunger turned into satisfaction. In addition to feeling surprisingly satisfied on so few calories during their Power Burn Days, test panelists told us again and again that their food cravings vanished within a few days of starting the 2 Day Diabetes Diet. Gone was the need to battle that crazy desire for extra between-meal snacks, sweets at night, salty or crunchy or sugary goodies in times of stress. As one dieter said, "Once you get started, your body gets used to the change. It really works."

Put an end to cheats and binges. You might worry whether you can handle the Power Burn Days—but you will surprise yourself! When studying these kinds of diets, some researchers assumed their patients would compensate and binge on their non-"fasting" days. But researchers have repeatedly found that's not true: Even when people are allowed to eat whatever they want the day after their "fast," they tend to eat only about 10 percent more calories, certainly not enough to offset the calorie deficit of the Power Burn Days.

After a few days of growling stomachs, as people remain on the program, they find they are able to be more easily satisfied with less food. Their leptin resistance resets itself; their insulin levels normalize. Their whole body is restored to factory settings, hormone doing its job to help them feel fuller faster, enjoy healthy and delicious food again in the most satisfying way possible, and shed pounds quickly.

By sticking with a few tough days in the beginning of the program, not only will your body get stronger—your mind will as well. Willpower is like a muscle—every time you resist something, your ability to withstand the temptation gets stronger. (That being said, if you feel nauseated or faint on your Power Burn days, stop and check your blood sugar. Also, try the tips in the box on page 49; if these don't help, eat a little more.)

How to Stay True to the Plan

Try these tips to boost your self-control.

Keep treats out of sight and out of mind. A study of office workers found that those who kept candy in their drawer instead of on their desk ate less.

Make a plan. Creating a list of scenarios will help you resist the cookie tray. "If I go to the pizzeria, I'll order a salad," or "If I go to the Super Bowl party, I'll bring my meatless chili—that will fill me up."

Key into your motivation. Maybe you want to get off your medication. Maybe you want to look great at your 25th high school reunion—or your 40th. Maybe you simply want to live long enough to watch your grandchildren grow up. "He who has a why can endure any how." Keeping this quote from Nietzsche in mind can really help get you through your next tussle with a platter of nachos.

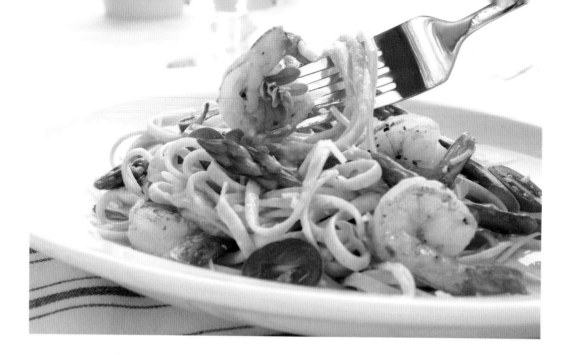

Practice #2: Nourishment Eating

On the 2 Day Diabetes Diet, when you are not power burning, you are nourishing.

Registered dietitian Erin Palinski-Wade developed Nourishment Days based on the eating style enjoyed for centuries by people who live on the shores of the Mediterranean Sea—in Italy, Greece, Crete, Spain, and other locales. Like their well-loved cuisine, Nourishment Days on the 2 Day Diabetes Diet are packed with fruit, vegetables, whole grains, fish, olive oil, nuts, seeds, and legumes. Main dishes feature lean proteins such as poultry as well as some eggs, cheese, and lean beef.

Nourishment Days are rich in fruits, vegetables, legumes, and other fiber-rich foods. All told, you'll enjoy 25 to 30 grams of appetite-suppressing dietary fiber daily on the 2 Day Diabetes Diet's Nourishment Days. That automatically moves you into the "ideal fiber intake" category—and ahead of the crowd when it comes to better blood sugar control. Most people just don't get enough produce or whole grains to hit these important levels. Fewer than 1 in 3 of us gets 2 or more servings of fruit and 3 servings of vegetables daily, according to the Centers for Disease Control. And just 1 in 12 gets 3 whole-grain servings a day![7]

Nourishment Days are also rich in dairy, which, a growing body of research is finding, can help you shed fat faster. This food group is rich in an array of nutrients—calcium, vitamin D, and protein—that shifts your body into fat-burning mode. An assortment of healthful fats from fish, nuts, olives, and more rounds out your Nourishment Days.

All told, your Nourishment Days will help you to nourish:

Blood sugar. Eating the mix of foods provided on Nourishment Days is your ticket to blood sugar success. In a 2011 study from Australia's University of Canberra, 27 people with well-controlled type 2 diabetes followed a Mediterranean way of eating (the same type of eating programmed into your Nourishment Days) for 12 weeks and then followed a standard healthy eating plan for another 12 weeks. Compared with the "usual" diet, the Mediterranean plan lowered average A1c levels (a check of long-term blood sugar control over 2 to 3 months) from 7.1 percent to a healthier 6.8 percent. Why the improvement? Study volunteers' blood levels of saturated fat and trans fatty acids—both of which can worsen the body's ability to obey signals from insulin, the hormone that tells cells to take in blood sugar—fell. And levels of monounsaturated fatty acids, shown in some studies to improve the way the body processes blood sugar, rose.[8]

> When you are not power burning, you are nourishing.

In another study, published in the *Journal of the Archives of Internal Medicine,* the Mediterranean diet reversed metabolic syndrome in more than 13 percent of participants over a year's time, while only 2 percent of participants achieved the same result following a low-fat diet.[9]

Finally, in a study by The Diabetes Clinic at Italy's Second University of Naples, the healthy fats, bountiful fiber, and rainbow of nutrients in the Mediterranean diet delayed the need for drugs. For 4 years, scientists tracked 215 overweight people newly diagnosed with type 2 diabetes who had never received diabetes medications. Half were assigned to eat a Mediterranean diet, while the other half followed a healthy low-fat diet. On both plans, women ate about 1,500 calories daily and men ate about 1,800. After 4 years, 4 percent of study volunteers on the Mediterranean diet needed diabetes medications for blood sugar control, compared to 7 percent of those who followed the low-fat diet.[10]

Weight loss. Yes, it sounds decadent, but this mix of foods will actually help you to slim down faster. When Israeli researchers compared three weight-loss plans—the Mediterranean diet, a low-carb diet, and a low-fat diet—the Mediterranean diet came out on top. At first, those in the low-carb and Mediterranean groups lost similar amounts of weight, but after 6 years the Mediterranean diet surged ahead, with Mediterranean dieters dropping an average of 7 pounds and keeping them off, compared to the low-carb group's 4 pounds. Why? Participants had an easier time staying on the Mediterranean diet long term. Due to its wide variety of options, participants were less likely to binge, cheat, quit, and relapse.[11]

Here's another possibility: The Mediterranean diet is rich in a particular type of fat called monounsaturated fatty acids (or MUFAs). Research from the Harvard Nurse's Health Study, one of the largest and longest-running studies in the world, found that this fat did not cause weight gain, but that saturated animal fat and trans fat (a human-made fat found in fried and processed foods) did.[12]

It's no wonder that British researchers who pioneered the 2 day diet concept chose to pair their 2 low-calorie days per week with 5 days of luscious Mediterranean eating! As you'll recall, women in that stunning 2011 study who ate low-carbohydrate, low-calorie meals 2 days a week and then ate Mediterranean-style 5 days a week lost more weight and more body fat than those who counted calories 7 days a week.

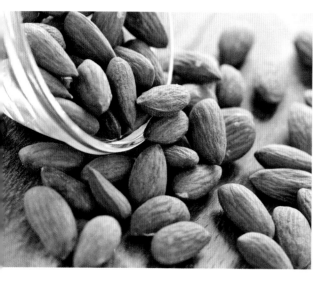

Satisfaction. Your Nourishment Days are rich in luscious fats, especially olive oil and nuts. Olive oil in particular might help induce a feeling of fullness between meals. As part of a study led by researchers from the Technische Universität München and the University of Vienna, study participants ate yogurt infused with either lard, butterfat, rapeseed oil, or olive oil every day. Those who consumed the olive oil–infused yogurt had higher concentrations of satiety hormones in their blood than participants who consumed the other oils. The olive oil consumers also reported more satisfaction.[13]

Lean protein, another feature of the Nourishment Days, also helps to fill you up and reduce hunger. And your Nourishment Days' heavy emphasis on heavy, water-rich, low-calorie fruits and vegetables helps to weigh down the stomach and induce a feeling of fullness.

Health. The Mediterranean diet is one of the most studied diets in the world, and the results are 100 percent positive. A study published in the *New England Journal of Medicine* found that the diet dropped deadly heart attack and stroke risk by 30 percent.[14] A different study from the *Journal of Clinical Endocrinology and Metabolism* found that the diet protected against bone loss.[15]

THE BETTER SEX DIET?

Could the food on your plate improve your passion and fun between the sheets? Researchers from Italy's Second University of Naples say the answer is yes, yes, yes. In a pair of studies published in 2010 in the *Journal of Sexual Medicine,* they looked at food choices and sexual function in 1,050 women and men with type 2 diabetes, ages 35 to 70. Since erectile dysfunction and a diminishment of sexual pleasure are realities for many with diabetes, these results may be especially important to you.

▸ Men who consumed nuts, fish, olive oil, and other foods that we promote on the Nourishment Days were about 1 percent less likely to have erectile dysfunction compared to those who did not.[16] They were also more likely to be sexually active.

▸ Women who most closely followed a Mediterranean diet were also about 1 percent less likely to be bothered by sexual problems such as trouble with lubrication, sensation, and orgasm. Like the men, they were also more likely to enjoy intimacy regularly.[17]

Practice #3: Satisfaction Eating

A small cookie . . . a glass of wine . . . or a square of delicious dark chocolate? On 2 of your 5 Nourishment Days each week on the 2 Day Diabetes Diet, you get to choose one of these treats, in addition to your snack for the day. Other options include light beer, a cocktail made with a sugar-free mixer, ice cream, baked chips, or one-half of a scone. We've crunched the numbers for you, so you can enjoy these snacks without guilt. They won't fill out your middle, and some of them—ice cream, wine, and chocolate—

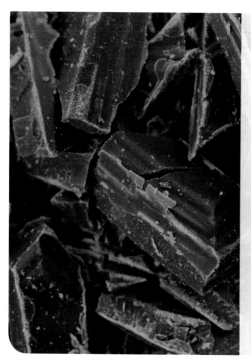

contain health-promoting ingredients that are even good for you! Here's how satisfying treats can ensure your success.

Stoke willpower. The Power Burn Days can be challenging, but knowing that you have a treat waiting for you during your Nourishment Days might help you over the more challenging humps. No matter how old we are, our brains never truly outgrow the sense of reward we get when we are promised a "treat." The neurochemical dopamine—the hormone of motivation—is triggered whenever we have the expectation of reward, whether that be a gold star from the teacher or a lollipop from the nice lady at the bank for being so well-behaved. Parents and teachers have long exploited this propensity for bribery to extract our good behavior—so now it's our turn to use it on ourselves.

Manage cravings. At a recent Endocrine Society annual meeting, researchers from Tel Aviv University presented findings from their study on 200 obese adults. Two groups were assigned to low-calorie diet programs. Both plans included breakfasts with lots of protein—fish, egg whites, cheese, and low-fat milk. But one plan added a sweet treat every day—chocolate!—that took the participants' breakfasts up to 600 calories.

Halfway through the study, both groups were doing great—they'd lost an average of 33 pounds. But by the end of the study, they'd parted ways—the low-carb group had regained 22 pounds each, but the sweet treat crew had shed an extra 15 pounds. After 32 weeks, the treaters were down an average of 40 pounds more than their low-carb compatriots. Not only did the breakfast feasters tap their body's higher morning metabolism, they also helped teach their bodies how to better regulate the hunger hormone ghrelin that we mentioned in Chapter 1, so it became easier to manage their appetites throughout the day.[20]

Boost blood sugar control and overall health. The treats offered on the 2 Day Diabetes Diet might seem decadent, but many of them are actually good for you. Ice cream, for instance, is rich in calcium and a special milk fat called trans-palmitoleic acid, thought to reduce risk for diabetes. People who consume more of this fat tend to have lower levels of inflammation and insulin, studies show. Other healing treats include red wine (which contains polyphenols thought to control blood sugar), beer and liquor (both heart protective), and dark chocolate (which contains flavonoids to reduce insulin resistance). Just remember that there is such a thing as too much of a good thing, so stick to the portions in our plan.

Practice #4: Tension Taming

Practice #4 is an optional component of the 2 Day Diabetes Diet, but it will go a long way to ensuring your success. We recommend you incorporate it into your Power Burn Days.

In Chapter 10, you'll find an assortment of Tension Tamers. These calming exercises do more than help you feel serene. Research shows that cultivating calm also gives your weight-loss and blood sugar control efforts a powerful boost.

Your calming practice will help you to:

Drop blood sugar. A landmark 2002 Duke University study was among the first to link stress reduction with better blood sugar numbers.

In this study, 108 women and men with type 2 diabetes got stress management training or took a diabetes class that didn't cover stress reduction. A year later, more than half of the stress-busting group saw blood sugar levels improve dramatically. Their A1c levels, a test of long-term blood sugar control, fell by 0.5 percent. And one in three saw A1c results drop by a full percentage point or more.[21,22]

Normalize cortisol. As we've mentioned, chronic overproduction of the stress hormone cortisol can produce other effects over time. For one thing, it triggers your body to store fat, making it harder to lose weight even if you're not overeating. To make matters worse, cortisol particularly stimulates fat storage in the belly area! Our Tension Tamers will halt the emotional stress that raises cortisol, so levels will drop down to normal.

Halve diabetes risk. Stress doesn't necessarily stem from difficult life events such as a job loss or caretaking of a loved one. Rather it arises out of your reaction to those events, which is why your Tension Taming plan is so important. It will help you to remain calm in the midst of crisis, something that is very important for stopping diabetes in its tracks. When Swedish researchers followed the heath outcomes of 7,500 men for 35 years, they came to a startling realization: stress nearly doubles your risk of developing diabetes. For the study, men were asked to grade their stress levels using a 6-point scale. Men who reported permanent stress—consistently high rankings on the scale during one or more years—had a 45 percent greater risk of developing type 2 diabetes by the end of the study compared to men who either had no stress or periodic stress. This increased risk was true regardless of age, income, physical fitness, and body weight.[23]

Defeat stress eating. Stress has a tendency to drive us straight to one place: the fridge. And it causes us to crave the very foods we're trying to limit: crunchy chips, sweet desserts, and other high-calorie fare. As we've mentioned, there's room on the 2 Day Diabetes Diet for indulgence, but stress makes it difficult to keep indulgence in check. That's precisely why we encourage you to do the Tension Tamers on Power Burn Days. With their low calories and carbs, Power Burn Days test your willpower more than the more robust and sumptuous Nourishment Days. Your Tension Tamers will help you pass that test with flying colors.

Drop more weight. Slashing stress can also help you lose weight and keep it off. In one 2008 study, researchers from New Zealand's Otago University found that women who learned stress management strategies lost weight—5 ½ pounds—while those who didn't tame tension didn't shed any pounds.[24] The stress-busters practiced muscle relaxation and breathing exercises similar to those selected for the 2 Day Diabetes Diet.

Practice #5: Moving

On the 2 Day Diabetes Diet, exercise is also optional. That said, we highly encourage it. You'll get faster results—burn more calories, torch more body fat (especially belly fat), reduce your blood sugar levels, and build more sexy, sugar-sipping muscle.

In Chapter 11, you'll find a doable walking plan, along with a strength-training program. The results you'll see and feel will amaze you. Your clothes will fit better. You'll feel more energetic. You (and your family and friends) may even notice that your moods are brighter than ever. But on the inside, exercise quietly yet dramatically changes things for the better in profound ways. If you think of activity as a sponge that helps soak up excess sugar that's circulating around your system, you realize how important it is to get moving. Study after study shows that being active for 30 to 45 minutes on most days of the week is a key strategy for losing weight and helping control your blood sugar. Your optional exercise plan can help you to:

> Activity is a sponge that helps soak up excess sugar.

Cool inflammation. When you exercise moderately, as the 2 Day Diabetes Diet suggests, your muscles produce anti-inflammatory substances that inhibit inflammation throughout your body.

Slash high blood sugar. In one amazing 2012 study from Maastricht University in the Netherlands, people with diabetes who exercised at a moderate pace for a half-hour just 3 to 4 days a week slashed their exposure to the damaging effects of high blood sugar by 2 percent.[25] The researchers found that while nonexercisers' blood sugar levels spiked to high levels nearly 8 hours each day, exercisers' blood sugar levels stayed in a healthy range almost 3 hours longer every day—a difference that lowered their long-term risk for diabetes-related complications like nerve damage, vision loss, and kidney problems.

Lose more weight. In a 2011 study from Seattle's Fred Hutchinson Cancer Research Center, women who followed a healthy, reduced-calorie diet and exercised regularly lost an average of 19.8 pounds in a year. In contrast, those who only exercised lost an average of 4.4 pounds and those who only dieted lost 15.8 pounds.[25]

Melt more belly fat. In a 2006 Johns Hopkins University study, 104 women and men who walked on a treadmill or rode exercise bikes 3 days a week and did a strength-training routine lost 18 percent of their belly fat.[27] This combination beats walking alone. In a 2010 study published in the *International Journal of Sport Nutrition and Exercise Metabolism*, women who walked and performed a simple strength-training routine 3 days a week slimmed their midsections 2 percent more than those who just walked.[28]

Nourish the Pounds Off—For Life!

Have you ever lost weight only to regain it all again? It's a common and frustrating experience.

We've taken every precaution to make sure this diet is your last diet. During all levels of the diet, you'll enjoy delicious, satisfying meals with high nutritional content. As a result, the 2 plus 5 approach is your secret to losing all the weight you want. Then, once you reach your goal, you'll follow Nourishment Days all 7 days a week. That's because research shows that the healthful fats, lean proteins, and delectable treats showcased on Nourishment Days are just what you need for lasting weight loss. And, on the off chance you do regain, just switch back to 2 plus 5 eating until you're back to your goal.

We're convinced that this will be the most effective diet you've ever tried, as well as the last one you ever start. Turn to Chapter 4 to find out why it will also be the most delicious.

THE 2 DAY WAY
Annette Sweeney

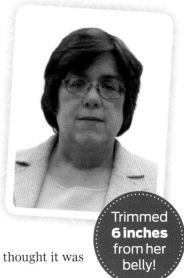

Trimmed **6 inches** from her belly!

Bankers aren't known for taking risks—at least in this economy! And banking executive Annette Sweeney is no different than most. She did her due diligence before she signed on the 2 Day dotted line. "Starting the diet was very difficult for me," says the 55-year-old. "It was hard to wrap my mind around the details. But once I figured out what I could make work in my life with commuting and getting home late, it all started to come together. And as tough as I thought it was going to be, I ended up finding it entirely manageable."

Annette, who is at risk for diabetes, received an amazing return on her investment: She lost 14 ½ pounds and 6 inches from her waist after 6 weeks on the diet. "I've had much more success on this diet than any of the other weight-loss plans I've tried in the last 10 years," she says. "The Power Burn Days were the most restrictive I've been on—which makes it all the more interesting that I've been able to stick with it, even through diet disaster times like Halloween, Thanksgiving, and Hurricane Sandy!"

The key to the 2 Day, Annette's way:

> ▶ **She did her research before she dove in.** "Once I understood the underpinnings of the diet, I could see how keeping it simple and balanced could really work," says Annette. "I could see how a turkey sandwich at lunch would be much more satisfying—and therefore much more conducive to diet success—than just a big salad."
>
> ▶ **She strategized to survive the second Power Burn Day.** "I wasn't typically hungry on the first Power Burn Day of the week," says Annette, "but by the second one, I was at first. I drank as much water as I could and stretched out the food for that day to allow for snacking at different intervals throughout the day."
>
> ▶ **She committed to making the plan a lifetime habit.** While she found the plan a little complicated at first, Annette notes, "It worked and it worked quickly. It's definitely something that can be fit into one's lifestyle [if you] find the days that you like and that you can fit into your routine."

CHAPTER 4

The Foods
of the 2 Day Diabetes Diet

Delicious real foods are the foundation of good health. These powerfully slimming foods will help balance your blood sugar and keep you satisfied.

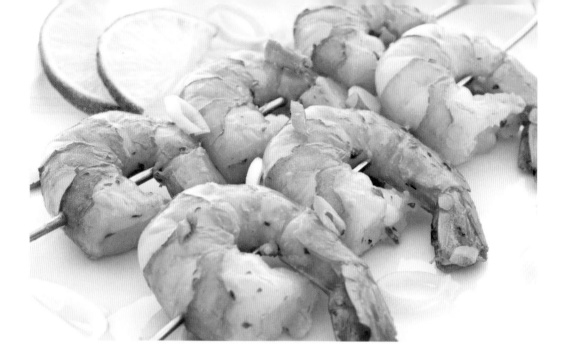

Dig into a Mushroom Quiche (page 173) or whole-grain waffle for breakfast, a lunchtime Pita Pizza topped with melted mozzarella and Gryuère cheese (page 223), or Spinach-Stuffed Meat Loaf (page 199) for dinner—and even savor goodies like dark chocolate, a cookie or scone, or a glass of beer or wine twice a week. On the 2 Day Diabetes Diet, every meal and snack is fresh, flavorful, and satisfying.

But beneath all that tasty goodness is a brilliant storehouse of powerful foods—all research-proven to maximize insulin sensitivity, decrease blood sugar levels, cool inflammation, and heal many of the problems that may have led to your diabetes in the first place.

You'll fill each plate with the healthiest (and yummiest!) foods nature has to offer.

No matter whether you are power burning or nourishing, you'll fill each plate with the healthiest (and yummiest!) foods nature has to offer. The fiber from whole grains, the satisfying fats from olives and avocados, the stick-to-your-ribs proteins in chicken and other lean meats, and the delectable calcium from cheese and other dairy products work together to turn down hunger and cravings while keeping your taste buds singing. Trust us: You won't feel deprived.

In addition to this wonderful cornucopia of foods and food groups, you'll zero in on fourteen diabetes superfoods and four diabetes super seasonings have been worked into many of the Power Burn and Nourishment Day meals, snacks, and recipes. They include blueberries, broccoli, cannellini beans, collard greens, fish, hot peppers, mushrooms, olive oil and grapeseed oil, quinoa, pysllium husk, spinach, steel-cut oats, sweet potatoes, and walnuts. For best results, you'll consume a superfood and a super seasoning at least three times a week. Look for "Superfood Spotlight" features throughout this book to learn more about each of these amazing foods.

Let's take a closer look into how specific foods fit into the 2 Day Diabetes Diet to help you achieve lasting success.

Power Burn Foods

We've created an absolutely satisfying menu of foods and snacks for your 2 weekly Power Burn Days to keep you feeling full and energized. If you take a look at the number of servings of various types of foods you will be consuming on these low-calorie, low- carb days, we think you'll be surprised. Two servings of fruit? Two servings of milk? A half serving of starch? Yes indeed, on this plan you can still consume these soul-satisfying food groups—even on your low-carb Power Burn Days. Erin went the extra mile to work them into your plan.

Now don't let our numbers confuse you. On this plan you do not need to count servings or points or anything unless you want to. We're just giving you the details so you have an idea of the overall daily goals. On Levels 1 and 2 of this diet, we've done the work of calculating and combining the right foods with the optimal combination of nutrients into ready-made meal options. In Level 3, you have the flexibility of creating your own menus. By matching your food choices to the number of servings listed, you can make nearly any meal a Power Burn meal.

Now, what will you be eating on your Power Burn Days? Here's what those servings look like on your plate: How about Canadian bacon and spinach for

POWER BURN DAYS
(2 DAYS A WEEK)

Here's what you'll be eating on each of the 2 Power Burn Days:

- ▸ 4 servings of vegetables
- ▸ 2 servings of fruit
- ▸ ½ serving of whole grains and other starches
- ▸ 3 ounces of lean protein
- ▸ 1 serving of good fats
- ▸ 2 servings of low-fat dairy
- ▸ 8 ounces of bouillon

breakfast with a cup of milk; vegetable soup and half a banana topped with peanut butter for lunch; grilled chicken and zucchini over pasta for dinner; and an orange with a cup of milk for a snack? With real, delicious food filling your tummy, you won't believe it all adds up to only 600 calories.

And the beautiful part? When you're done with those 2 days, you can delight 5 days a week in bountiful quantities of delicious, stick-to-your-ribs meals—meat and fish and potatoes, fresh bread and crunchy salads and yogurts, fruits, even chocolate, wine, and pasta! No wonder so many of our participants proclaimed the 2 Day Diabetes Diet "the last diet I'll ever need"—anyone could easily stay on this plan for life, with very few modifications.

Nourishment Foods

During the 5 Nourishment Days of the week, you'll follow a delicious 1,500-calorie-a-day eating plan, which Erin developed using the nutritional framework of the research-proven Mediterranean diet. As mentioned earlier, the Mediterranean diet follows the traditional eating plan of people who live in Italy, Greece, and other countries bordered by the Mediterranean Sea. People of this region eat lots of fruits, vegetables, whole grains, fish, olive oil, nuts, seeds and legumes, poultry, eggs and cheese, herbs, and spices. They eat fewer servings of red meat and sweets, and very few processed, packaged, fast, or junk foods. They're also active and drink red wine in moderation.

Research has found that people who follow this lifestyle have a lower risk for heart disease, cancer, and other chronic diseases than do people who eat a typical Western-style diet. What's more, this diet is proven to help you control blood sugar and maintain a healthy weight—for life.

We've adapted this healthy diet for the Nourishment Days of the 2 Day Diabetes Diet program.

THE NOURISHMENT DAYS
(5 DAYS PER WEEK)

Here's what you'll be eating on each of the 5 Nourishment Days:

▶ 4 servings of vegetables

▶ 2 servings of fruit

▶ 5 servings of whole grains and other starches

▶ 10 ounces of lean protein

▶ 5 servings of good fats

▶ 2 servings of low-fat dairy

While all the meals follow the same nutritional Mediterranean profile, with plenty of fruits, vegetables, whole grains, and healthy fats, eating according to the guidelines of the Mediterranean diet doesn't mean you're limited to Mediterranean flavors. You'll enjoy a bounty of brightly colored fruits and vegetables, lean proteins, whole grains, and even a few treats. You'll savor Grilled Chicken Kabobs (page 204) with pasta, or dig into delicious Honey-Lime Pork Chops (page 203) with Tex-Mex Red Beans (page 244) for dinner (which our 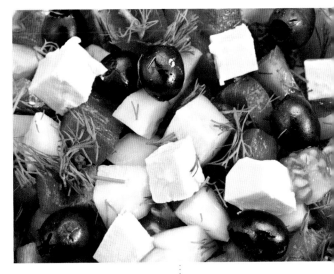 test panelists just loved!). How about Baked Sweet Potato "Fries" (page 238), sautéed collard greens, or elegant Roasted Asparagus and Red Pepper with Parmesan (page 234)?

Does it seem too good to be true? It's not. Let's take a closer look.

Powerfully Slimming Foods

How on earth could this delicious assortment of foods still be so great for weight control? This plan's luscious fats and healthy yet satisfying proteins will fill you up and keep you feeling full. Produce and whole grains go even further to fill you up (but not out) and prevent food cravings. Many of these foods boast health-promoting vitamins, minerals, antioxidants, and other phytonutrients that switch on healthy genes that promote weight loss and switch off the genes that can contribute to excess pounds. Let's take it step-by-step and break down each facet of the 2 Day Diabetes Diet eating plan, so you can fully appreciate the nutritional powerhouse this diet really is.

2 DAY DIABETES DIET SUPERFOODS

These delectable foods and spices work powerfully to improve diabetes and prevent complications. Enjoying these at least three times per week—and ideally, every day—can help power up your weight loss and power down your blood sugar. We've worked these into your 2 Week Quick Start Meal Plan, as well as into the additional meal options—and eliminated the guesswork! To learn more about these antidiabetes superfoods, look for "Superfood Spotlight" features throughout the book.

Blueberries	Collard greens	Quinoa
Broccoli	Fish	Spinach
Cannellini beans	Hot peppers	Steel-cut oats
Cayenne pepper	Mushrooms	Sweet potatoes
Cinnamon	Olive oil or grapeseed oil	Turmeric
Cloves	Psyllium husk	Walnuts

Vegetables

Servings per Nourishment Day: 4
Servings per Power Burn Day: 4

Arugula	Chives	Onions
Beets	Collard greens	Peppers
Bok choy	Eggplant	Rutabaga
Broccoli	Kale	Shallots
Broccoli rabe	Kohlrabi	Spinach
Brussels sprouts	Leeks	Summer squash
Cabbage	Lettuce (Bibb, buttercrunch, Romain)	Tomato
Carrots		Turnip greens
Cauliflower	Mustard greens	Watercress

On Power Burn Days and Nourishment Days, you'll find a rainbow of colors and flavors of Mother Nature's goodies. As you've probably heard, vegetables are incredibly good for you. In the plant world, the pigments that make vegetables green, red, purple, orange, and yellow double as disease fighters. In plants, these disease fighters fend off rot, insects, and other problems. In our bodies, these same disease fighters protect our cells from cancer. One of the nutrients that gives vegetables their rich color, for instance, is beta-carotene, a precursor of vitamin A. The deep green of kale, the bright orange of sweet potatoes and pumpkin, and the brilliant red of red bell peppers all reveal the presence of this powerful health promoter, which is essential for a healthy immune system and healthy skin and eyes.

Another wonder nutrient in plants, especially green leafy ones, is lutein. This pigment is great for protecting your eyesight, which is good news because people who are prone to developing diabetes are also prone to vision problems.

But here's how vegetables help with what you're most concerned about: blood sugar problems and stubborn fat.

Vegetables balance your blood sugar long term. The salads, spinach, collards, and other greens you'll find on this meal plan serve an important purpose. Leafy veggies are tops at reducing risk for developing type 2 diabetes since they are rich in nutrients such as magnesium and vitamin K, which have been linked to a decreased risk of diabetes and improved blood sugar control. A study by the Centers for Disease Control and Prevention found that people who ate 5 servings of fruits and veggies every day cut their risk of developing full-blown diabetes within 2 decades by 20 percent compared with people who didn't eat any. This effect was especially strong for women, and researchers found this strong link even after controlling for age, race or ethnicity, cigarette smoking, blood pressure, cholesterol, BMI, exercise levels, and alcohol use.[1]

And in a 2012 study from Japan's Shikoku University of 417 people with diabetes, those who ate the most vegetables had the lowest and healthiest A1c levels (a check of long-term blood sugar levels).[2] How much were they eating? The study, published in the journal *Geriatrics and Gerontology International,* found that the biggest veggie munchers consumed about 1½ cups total of vegetables a day, including about a half-cup of green types like spinach, green beans, and broccoli. That's a goal you'll easily meet by following the 2 Day Diabetes Diet's food plans.

Produce is blood sugar friendly for several reasons. First, it's full of fiber, which slows down digestion after a meal and can help prevent spikes in blood sugar levels. Vegetables and most fruits are considered naturally low in carbohydrates, too, and what carbohydrate they do contain is packed with water. End result: These foods contain very few carbs and calories. Second, produce contains several nutrients that help cool off chronic inflammation—which, as you might remember from Chapter 1, is a condition that worsens insulin resistance so that your cells have trouble absorbing and burning blood sugar.

Vegetables satisfy you with few calories. Full of fiber and water yet low in calories, vegetables are what weight-loss experts call "high-volume, low-energy-density" foods. Translation: They take up a lot of space in your stomach (and take a while to chew!), so you fill up without filling out, according to a 2010 University of Arizona review of produce and weight-control research published in the journal *Obesity Reviews*.[3]

Vegetables allow you to eat more food. Adding produce was better for weight loss than simply cutting out high-fat, high-calorie foods in one 2007 Pennsylvania State University study, published in the *American Journal of Clinical Nutrition*. The researchers followed the diets and weights of 71 volunteers, and after a year, those whose reduced-calorie diets included more fruits and veggies lost 17 ½ pounds, compared to about 14 pounds for those who simply cut calories. The fruit and veggie group downed about 1 to 2 cups of produce per day. They reported less hunger than the fat-slashing group, perhaps because the produce group actually ate 2 percent more food by weight![4]

Vegetables reduce heart disease. People with diabetes are at an increased risk for heart disease and stroke, and piling your plate with produce can lower your risk for a heart attack or stroke by 30 percent.[5] Why? Soluble fiber, such as pectin, in many types of vegetables helps your body eliminate LDL ("bad") cholesterol by binding with cholesterol-rich bile acids in your digestive system so you literally "flush" cholesterol away. As part of a healthy diet, produce delivers minerals like potassium, magnesium, and calcium that help keep blood pressure lower and healthier.

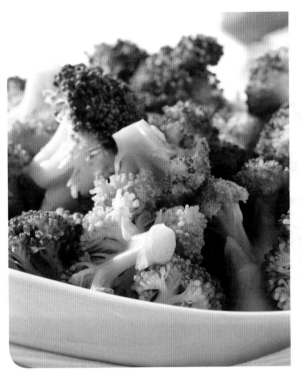

SUPERFOOD SPOTLIGHT: Broccoli

Broccoli is an antidiabetes superhero. It and other cruciferous veggies like kale and cauliflower contain a compound called sulforaphane, which triggers a whole host of anti-inflammatory processes that improve blood sugar control and protect blood vessels from the cardiovascular damage that's often a consequence of diabetes. (Heart disease is the leading cause of death for people with diabetes, so this protection could be a lifesaver!) Sulforaphane also helps flip on the body's natural detox mechanisms, helping enzymes turn dangerous cancer-causing chemicals into more innocent forms that the body can easily release.

Fruit

Servings per Nourishment Day: 2

Servings per Power Burn Day: 2

Apples	Grapefruit	Papayas
Apricots	Grapes	Peaches
Bananas	Honeydew	Pears
Berries	Kiwifruits	Pineapple
Blackberries	Lemons	Plums
Blueberries	Limes	Raspberries
Cantaloupe	Mangoes	Starfruits
Cherries	Melon	Strawberries
Clementines	Nectarines	Watermelon
Figs	Oranges	

Extreme low-carbohydrate diets skimp on fruit, because, they claim, fruit contains natural sugars that turn into sugar in the body. It's true that all carbohydrates from food eventually end up as blood glucose—including the carbs in fruit. That said, fruit has a much lower impact on blood sugar levels than other truly harmful foods like candy bars and soft drinks. That's because, like vegetables, fruit is mostly water. What isn't water is fiber, and that fiber slows the progression of fruit sugars into the bloodstream, causing a slow, steady rise in blood sugar rather than a huge spike.

Fruit isn't just not *bad* for your diabetes. It's good for it, and for your waistline, too.

Here's more: Fruit isn't just *not bad* for your diabetes. It's good for it, and for your waistline, too.

Fruit fights off inflammation. Peaches, plums, and nectarines contain special nutrients called phenolic compounds that have anti-inflammatory properties. These compounds travel through the bloodstream and then to your fat cells, where they affect different genes and proteins for the better, finds research done at Texas A&M University.[6]

Fruit prevents diabetes. Flavonoids are nutrients found in plant foods, and especially in many types of fruit. Research shows that these compounds can lower risk for developing type 2 diabetes, probably because these nutrients improve insulin sensitivity.[7] Harvard's long-running Nurses' Health Study found that women who consumed more anthocyanins (the pigment that makes blueberries blue and strawberries red) were much less likely to develop type 2 diabetes than women who consumed fewer of these health-promoting compounds.[8]

Fruit slims you down. New research suggests fruits may actually be more important than vegetables when it comes to long-term weight loss. A Utah State University study followed the eating habits of 77 overweight and obese people to see what effects fruit consumption would have on their weight. Months later, when the researchers crunched all the data, they determined that it was fruit that was the deciding factor in weight loss. The more fruit people ate, the more weight they lost.[9] This study is no anomaly. When a Danish team looked at all the available studies about fruit and body weight, they found that, out of 16 studies, two indicated that eating more fruit helps you lose weight; five found that eating more fruit reduces your risk of gaining weight or becoming obese; and four studies found the same inverse association as the Utah study—the more fruit you eat, the fewer pounds you weigh.[10]

Fruit bolsters health. Along with vegetables, fruit protects against heart disease, stroke, and cancers of the stomach and colon. It also helps fend off depression, which is common in people with diabetes.[11]

Sold? We sure hope so. One way to ensure you consume more fruit (and vegetables) is this: Shop local. Local produce—fresh, juicy, and full of sun-ripened flavor—is everywhere these days, thanks to the increasing popularity of farmers' markets, backyard gardens, and community gardens. And this food trend can motivate you to eat more produce, reaping big weight-control and health benefits. Recent research shows that the experience of growing produce or shopping at a farmstand inspires people to eat more fruits and vegetables.[12] If you're among the many adults who aren't eating the U.S. Department of Agriculture's recommended 2 to 2 ½ cups of vegetables and 1½ to 2 cups of fruit a day, getting up close and personal with your produce could help.

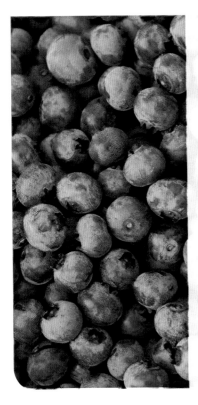

SUPERFOOD SPOTLIGHT: Blueberries

Some fruits house so much nutrition that they stand out from the pack. Blueberries are a prime example. They are packed with both insoluble fiber (the kind that bulks up stool and "flushes" fat out of your system) and soluble fiber (the kind that forms a gel in your intestine, slowing stomach emptying and improving blood sugar control). In a study by the USDA, people who consumed 2 ½ cups of wild blueberry juice per day for 12 weeks lowered their blood glucose levels, lifted depression, and improved their memories.[13] Researchers credit these results to blueberries' anthocyanins, a natural chemical that shrinks fat cells and also stimulates the release of adiponectin, a hormone that regulates blood glucose levels, among other things. Increasing adiponectin levels can help keep blood sugar low and increase our sensitivity to insulin.[14] Don't skimp on these gorgeous, sweet, satisfying natural candies. When they're in season, visit your local farmers' market and indulge! Eat them by the handful, and freeze them for the winter. Throw them into yogurt and smoothies, put them in salads, sprinkle them over oatmeal and cereal.

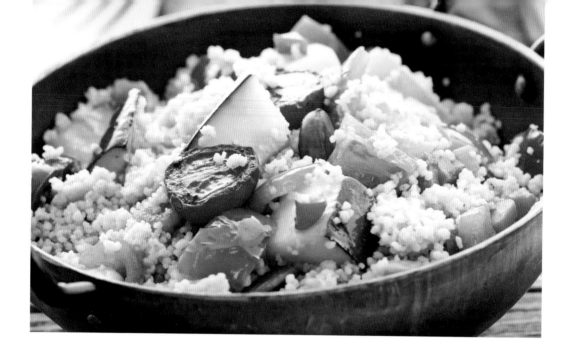

Whole Grains and Other Starches

Servings per Nourishment Day: 5

Servings per Power Burn Day: ½

Barley

Beans (such as black, cannellini, fava, garbanzo, great northern, kidney, lima, mung, navy, pink, pinto) and lentils*

Bean, whole-grain

Buckwheat

Bulgur

Corn**

Couscous

Millet

Oats (steel-cut preferred)

Pasta, whole-grain

Peas**

Popcorn

Pumpkin**

Rice, brown and wild

Quinoa

Sweet potato**

Wheat bran

Winter squash**

All beans contain both protein and starch, so we have listed them in both places.

**Although these are vegetables, because they are higher in carbohydrates and calories, they count as a starch for the purposes of the 2 Day Diabetes Diet meal plans.*

The greater abundance of calories and carbs on your Nourishment Days allows you to consume a hearty 5 servings of whole grains, but Erin made sure never to completely omit grains, even on your super low-calorie Power Burn Days. That's because she knew, from counseling so many clients over the years, just how important grains are to your overall success.

Crunchy granola. Hearty whole-grain breads. Tasty, easy-to-cook side dish grains like quinoa, bulgur, and whole-wheat couscous. Even whole-grain waffles. The grains on your plate during the 2 Day Diabetes Diet are true superfoods that taste great as they help you whittle your waist, control your blood sugar, and improve your health. The average American eats 6.7 ounces of grains a day, which is quite a bit of grain and more than 100 percent of what experts recommend. Here's the problem: More than three-quarters of those grains are refined, according to the US Department of Agriculture. For satisfaction and total body health, you want the reverse. In other words, most of your grains should be whole and only a tiny bit refined. That's exactly what the 2 Day Diabetes Diet promotes. Here's why whole grains are featured, especially on Nourishment Days, on our plan.

The grains on your plate during the 2 Day Diabetes Diet are true superfoods.

Whole grains improve insulin sensitivity and reduce risk of diabetes. Whole grains are loaded with soluble fiber, which helps control blood sugar. That's probably why eating 4 servings of whole grains daily reduced risk for developing prediabetes by 30 percent in a 2012 study from Sweden's Karolinska University.[15] In one University of South Carolina study of 978 people, whole grains improved insulin sensitivity, too.[16]

Whole grains reduce systemic inflammation. In a 2008 Pennsylvania State University study, whole-grain eaters also saw body-wide inflammation fall by 38 percent, which could reduce risk for insulin resistance, heart disease, and high blood pressure. In contrast, those who ate refined grain products saw no reduction in inflammation levels even though they had lost weight.[17] The researchers aren't sure why whole grains reduced inflammation, but note that whole-grain eaters took in more fiber and magnesium than those who munched refined grains.

Whole grains whittle your waist. Could the type of bread, rice, or pasta you choose affect your weight and waistline? Yes, it can. In the same

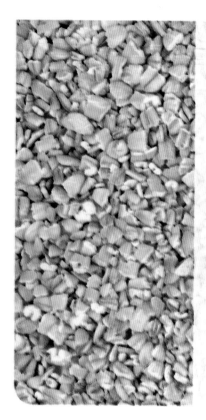

SUPERFOOD SPOTLIGHT: Steel-Cut Oats

You may not think of humble oatmeal as a superfood, but you might change your mind when you discover this piece of news: Eating oatmeal can help reduce the risk of developing type 2 diabetes. Turns out that oatmeal contains high amounts of magnesium, which helps the body to properly use glucose and secrete insulin. An 8-year trial showed a 19 percent decrease in type 2 diabetes risk in women with a magnesium-rich diet and a 31 percent decreased risk in women who regularly ate whole grains.[20]

Steel-cut oats are just as easy to cook as standard oatmeal, but they haven't been overly processed the way quick-cooking oats have. When grains are left whole, they have high amounts of resistant carbohydrates, which means they are filled with the fiber, nutrients, and bound antioxidants that give your body more of a digestive challenge, allowing blood sugar to remain more stable.

Even if you're a lifelong oatmeal lover, give steel-cut oats a try—they're heartier and chewier than traditional oatmeal, and they stick to the ribs, giving you more satisfaction for the calories.

Pennsylvania State University study we just mentioned, 50 extremely overweight volunteers followed a healthy, low-calorie diet for 12 weeks. One group ate refined carbohydrates such as white bread, white rice, and regular pasta while the other ate whole-grain products like whole-wheat bread and brown rice. While both groups lost 8 to 11 pounds, the whole-grain group lost significantly more abdominal fat—a change that meant not just trimmer physiques but better health.[18]

Whole grains slash the risk of heart disease. Heart disease is one of the most common complications of diabetes, and 2 to 3 whole-grain servings a day slashed risk for a heart attack or deadly heart disease by 30 percent in the landmark Nurses' Health Study.[19] Why? Grains rich in soluble fiber help whisk cholesterol out of the body.

Lean Protein

Servings per Nourishment Day: 10 ounces

Servings per Power Burn Day: 3 ounces

Beans (such as black, cannellini, fava, garbanzo, great northern, kidney, lima, mung, navy, pink, pinto, soy) and lentils*

Beef, lean (such as bottom round, sirloin, tenderloin, top round)

Cheese, low-fat (such as cheddar, cottage, mozzarella)

Eggs

Fish (such as cod, eel, halibut, sardine, snapper, salmon, tuna)

Game meat (such as buffalo, ostrich, venison)

Lamb, lean

Pork, lean (chops, tenderloin)

Poultry, skinless, white meat (such as chicken, duck, goose, turkey)

Shellfish (such as abalone, clam, crab, lobster, mussel, oyster, scallop, shrimp)

All beans contain both protein and starch, so we have listed them in both places.

**While cheese is a dairy product, because low-fat cheeses primarily contribute protein to your diet, for the purposes of the 2 Day Diabetes Diet meal plan, they count as a protein.*

Most North Americans eat plenty of protein, and Erin made sure to include a hearty dose on Nourishment Days to satisfy those meat-and-potato appetites. She also snuck a good chunk of protein into your super-low-calorie Power Burn Days, too. Your 3 ounces of protein on those days amounts to a serving of meat or fish that is roughly the size of a deck of cards. It will go a long way toward making Power Burn Days seem like any other day, and not the modified fast that they are.

Emerging research suggests that the type of protein you choose can make a difference in your health and even your weight. That's why this eating plan showcases lean protein such as chicken, lean cuts of pork and beef, and beans. You'll also get protein from your 2 daily servings of dairy and from the nuts and nut butters on the menu.

Protein levels are kept within a healthy range on the 2 Day Diabetes Diet. We've avoided the huge servings of meat found on some low-carb plans because excess protein is not recommended for the estimated 40 percent of people with diabetes who also have reduced kidney function.[21] The "just right" protein level of this plan (10 ounces on Nourishment Days and 3 ounces on Power Burn Days) delivers flavor, satisfaction, and the following host of deeper benefits.

Lean protein can reduce diabetes risk. Certain types of protein help improve insulin sensitivity, and other types work against it. This plan goes with the former (lean options) and nixes the latter (fatty options). (One exception to this rule, as you'll soon learn, is the fat in dairy products.) As it turns out, meats packed with saturated fat may make it more difficult for your body to readily absorb blood sugar. In a 2008 study from the University of Minnesota, people who ate fatty meats 2 times a day had a 25 percent higher risk for blood sugar problems than those who ate more lean proteins such as skinless poultry, fish, and beans.[22]

> The "just right" protein level delivers flavor, satisfaction, and a host of deeper benefits.

Slashing saturated fat helped people with prediabetes lower their risk for developing full-blown diabetes by 58 percent in the landmark Diabetes Prevention Program study, published in 2002 in *The New England Journal of Medicine*.[23] And in a 2007 University of Oklahoma study of 1,204 people with type 2 diabetes, those who ate the most saturated fat were 58 percent more likely to have poor blood sugar control than those who ate the least.[24]

Some lean proteins exert their own beneficial effect on blood sugar as well. For example, the white and red beans you'll enjoy on the 2 Day Diabetes Diet, in dishes like Tex-Mex Red Beans (page 244) and creamy cannellini beans, deliver blood sugar–lowering fiber. As you'll discover in our discussion of dairy products, milk and yogurt provide sugar-controlling nutrients, too. And the good fats in protein-rich nuts and fish are also shown to pamper your blood sugar.

Lean protein helps you burn fat and build muscle. Many dieters lose a combination of fat (what we all want to lose) and muscle (what we don't want to lose) as they drop pounds. Muscle is important not only because it powers your daily movements, but also because it burns calories round the clock. Even when you are not using it, muscle is busy, active tissue, constantly remodeling itself. This constant remodeling uses

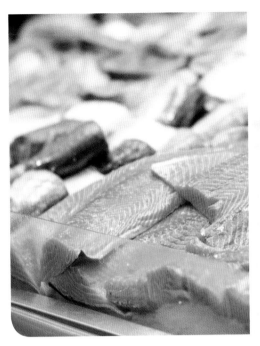

SUPERFOOD SPOTLIGHT: Fish

Fish is a slimming star for two reasons. One is that fish is rich in protein, which will help to keep you satisfied. Secondly, fish contains a special type of fat that helps cool inflammation. Thousands of studies show that people with the highest blood levels of omega-3 fatty acids have less body-wide inflammation, the very inflammation that leads to and worsens diabetes and weight problems. A fish-rich diet can also reduce your risk of developing health problems, especially stroke, as a result of your diabetes. People who ate baked, broiled, or steamed fish reduced their odds for a stroke by 3 percent, found a 2010 Emory University study.[27] (However, fried fish—such as fast-food fish sandwiches, fish sticks, and fried seafood of any type—increased risk.)

up a lot of calories, so every pound of muscle helps you lose weight. It also helps control blood sugar. As you can see, ideally, you want to preserve muscle as you drop pounds. Your 2 Day Diet exercise plan will help, but so will the lean protein on your plate. Getting enough protein helped 90 overweight women hold on to more lean muscle mass while dieting in one 2011 study from Canada's McMaster University, published in the *Journal of Nutrition*.[25]

Lean protein keeps you satisfied. Protein is certainly your best friend during the Power Burn Days of the 2 Day Diabetes Diet. Protein can help you feel fuller after a meal—and stay fuller longer than if you'd eaten a meal containing more carbs or fat, Harvard School of Public Health researchers report in a 2004 review in the *Journal of the American College of Nutrition*.[26]

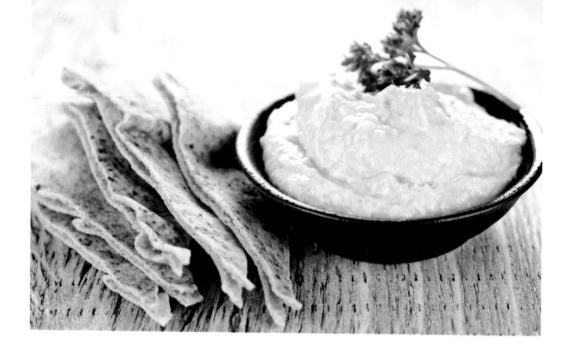

Good Fats

Servings per Nourishment Day: 3
Servings per Power Burn Day: 1

Almonds	Hummus	Pine nuts
Avocado	Macadamias	Pistachios
Brazil nuts	Olive oil or olive oil margarine	Pumpkin seeds
Cashews		Sesame seeds
Flaxseeds	Olives	Sunflower seeds
Guacamole	Pecans	Walnuts
Hazelnuts	Pesto	

You probably remember the low-fat diets that were all the rage in the 1980s and 1990s. Those diets restricted every single type of fat. End result: Many of us began consuming an abundance of foods that weren't good for our blood sugar levels at all, especially fat-free cookies and chips. And we stopped consuming many foods that were actually good for us because of the healthful fats housed inside.

We now know that many fatty foods—including olives, avocados, nuts, and vegetable oils—are not bad for us at all. Case in point: In the 1960s, when fats and oils accounted for 45 percent of dietary calories, only 13 percent of American adults were obese and less than 1 percent had type 2 diabetes. In the new millennium, Americans consume only 33 percent of their calories from fat, but now more than three times as many people are obese and 11 percent have diabetes, too.

As it turns out, the total amount of fat in our diets is much less important than the type of fat. Certain types of fat raise risk for diabetes and body fat; others drop risk.

TYPES OF FAT	COMMON FOODS	HOW THEY AFFECT HEALTH
Trans fats (also called partially hydrogenated fats)	Fried foods, baked goods, processed snack foods, and some margarines	Increase inflammation, worsen diabetes, hurt heart health
Saturated fats	Fatty animal products	May lead to insulin resistance and raise risk for certain types of cancer
Monounsaturated fats	Olive oil, peanuts, avocados, and certain types of nuts and seeds	Reduce insulin resistance, improve heart health, drop blood cholesterol and blood pressure
Omega-6 fats (a type of polyunsaturated fat)	Vegetable oils	Can increase inflammation when consumed in large amounts
Omega-3 fats (a type of polyunsaturated fat)	Fatty fish like salmon, chia seeds, and walnuts	Improve insulin sensitivity and heart health

Even on your Power Burn Days, Erin worked some fat into your plan. Whether you are nourishing or power burning, you'll maximize healthful fats and minimize harmful fats. This not only increases satisfaction (fat is what makes many foods worth eating), but it's also powerfully good for your weight and blood sugar. From pecans on your oatmeal to olive oil on your salad, the fats you eat on the 2 Day Diabetes Diet are types recognized by experts and proven in thousands of research studies to be tops for weight loss, blood sugar control, and all-around good health.

Good fats improve insulin sensitivity. When 162 people followed a diet full of monounsaturated fats, their insulin sensitivity improved by 9 percent, found a 2001 study from Sweden. In contrast, those who downed loads of saturated fat experienced a 12 percent decline in insulin sensitivity.[28] And in a Spanish study, people who ate plenty of these good fats at a single breakfast had better insulin sensitivity throughout the day than those who munched a morning meal rich in saturated fat or carbohydrates.[29]

Good fats can lower your A1c. Replacing the saturated fat in your diet (from fatty meats, butter, ice cream, and full-fat cheese, milk, and yogurt) with monounsaturated fat from nuts, olive oil, and avocado helps your body handle blood sugar in a healthier way—and does so quickly. In a 2011 study of 117 people with type 2 diabetes published in the journal *Diabetes Care,* University of Toronto researchers reported that replacing some carbohydrates with nuts lowered A1c levels. "Bad" LDL cholesterol levels also improved.[30]

Good fats whittle dangerous belly fat. Monounsaturated fats have also been shown in several studies to shrink belly fat. A good fat-rich diet reduces visceral fat while a high-carbohydrate, low-fat diet increases it, found a 2007 report from Spain's Reina Sofía University Hospital.[31]

Good fats spell satisfaction. If you've had trouble sticking with reduced-calorie diets in the past, here's good news: Adding good fats can help. Dieters were three times more likely to stay on a meal plan that contained plenty of monounsaturated fats than on a low-fat diet, found a 2001 study from Boston's Brigham and Women's Hospital.[32]

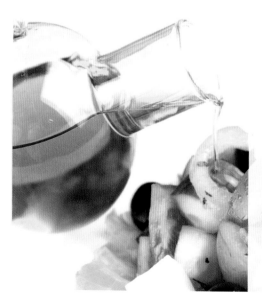

SUPERFOOD SPOTLIGHT: Olive Oil

Following a Mediterranean style of diet that is rich in olive oil helps to reduce the risk of type 2 diabetes by as much as 50 percent compared to a diet low in fat, finds a recent Spanish study.[33] And a different study done at Technical University of Munich (TUM) and the University of Vienna found that olive oil improved satiety the most when compared to lard, butter, and rapeseed oil.[34] In addition to being a standout source of health-promoting monounsaturated fats, olive oil is also rich in antioxidant nutrients that protect cells from damage and prevents the development of heart disease. Use it on salads and in place of butter.

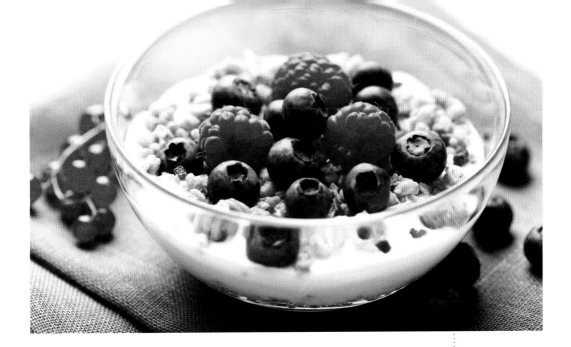

Dairy

Servings per Nourishment Day: 2

Servings per Power Burn Day: 2

Greek yogurt

Kefir

Low-fat yogurt, flavored
  (no sugar added)

Low-fat yogurt, plain

Milk, 2%

On the 2 Day Diabetes Diet, you'll enjoy dairy every day—in delicious, homemade smoothies, soups, and glasses of cool, refreshing milk.

If you take a look at the menus and recipes, however, you'll probably notice that, unlike many plans, we're not recommending skim and nonfat dairy options. No, we're recommending 2% milk. After so many years of being urged to drink skim milk in order to lose weight, is it a little bizarre to see 2% milk on this list? Not to worry—it's not a typo.

This is the type of milk used in the British study on which the 2 Day Diabetes Diet is based. It's a halfway point between skim and whole, but we went with 2% for another reason: Unlike the fats in other animal products, the fats in milk are actually good for you.

Cutting-edge research has begun to show that the type of saturated fat in dairy products is a powerful fat burner. A 2013 Swedish study followed almost 1,600 men between ages 40 and 60 for 12 years to see what impact dairy fat had on their waistlines. The results were shocking: Those men who had a lower than average intake of dairy fat at the beginning of the study (they ate no butter or low-fat milk, and they never ate whipped cream) had a higher risk of gaining belly fat than people who ate an average amount.[36] This difference held no matter how many fruits and vegetables the men ate, whether or not they smoked or drank, what they did for a living, even how much they exercised or how much they weighed at the start of the study. The researchers' conclusion: Dairy fat burns belly fat.

Dairy products contain two types of beneficial fats. One of them is called trans-palmitoleic acid, and it has been shown to drop diabetes risk by 60 percent. It also lowers insulin resistance.[37] Another, conjugated linoleic acid, is a fat that may help turn on the fat-burning process inside your body.

In addition to those fats, milk contains other nutrients that make it a good choice for people with diabetes. Let's take a closer look. (Note: If your digestive system can't handle cow's milk or you don't "do dairy" for other reasons, it's fine to substitute calcium-enriched soy milk or almond milk or to use milk formulated for people with lactose intolerance. See "I'm Lactose Intolerant. Can I Still Follow This Plan?" on page 84 for guidance.)

Dairy helps prevent insulin resistance. The calcium, magnesium, and vitamin D in dairy products help your body respond quickly to insulin, the hormone that tells cells that it's time to absorb blood sugar. That's important, because worsening insulin sensitivity is a major cause of type 2 diabetes. Harvard Medical School researchers have found that every daily dairy serving reduces risk for insulin resistance by 21 percent.[38] And researchers from France's National Institute of Health and Medical Research have found that people who consume 2 daily dairy servings are about 26 percent less likely to develop high blood sugar problems.[39]

Dairy helps you lose 30 percent more weight. Researchers from Iran's Isfahan University of Medical Sciences found that including reduced-fat dairy products—like those you'll enjoy on the 2 Day Diabetes Diet—helped dieters lose about 30 percent more weight.[40] The participants who consumed dairy lost more body fat, gained more lean body mass (muscle, bone, and other nonfat tissue), and trimmed their waistlines (a sign that they'd lost more deep abdominal fat) than those who had little or no dairy during weight loss. Wow![41]

Bouillon

Servings per Nourishment Days: Not required
Servings per Power Burn Day: 8 ounces

While it's certainly okay to sip bouillon during Nourishment Days, you'll definitely want to turn to it on Power Burn Days. That's when no-calorie liquids—from bouillon, water, tea, and other approved beverages—are most important. Your body will be quickly burning through its fuel stores on these days. When your body burns through that fuel, it releases water, and you must take several trips to the bathroom as a result.

It's incredibly important for you to stay hydrated as all of this fat burning is going on. A hormone called vasopressin increases when you're dehydrated, and this prompts your liver to produce more blood sugar.[42] Of course, staying hydrated also prevents you from overheating in warm weather or while exercising, which can also prompt blood sugar levels to rise.

Bouillon is a great way to prevent dehydration. It's one better than water because it's packaged with important electrolytes such as sodium that you'll also need to replace on Power Burn Days. Here are some other ways bouillon serves as a Power Burn Day darling.

Bouillon fills you up. Our bodies are very sophisticated machines, with lots of regulatory systems that help us balance our blood sugar levels and detect nutrients and use them to fight all kinds of diseases. However, when it comes to your stomach, it can be very easily outsmarted. When in doubt, all you need to do is think "volume." The higher the water content of our meals, the faster our stomachs fill up, and the faster we can be satisfied for the fewest number of calories. And what's the quick answer to how you can bring more water content into your mealtimes? Soup, soup, soup—all of it easily made from one of the simplest foods around: bouillon.

Bouillon can turn off hunger—without calories. If you are feeling a hunger pang between meals, just sip on some bouillon. Our test panelists told us that this was often all it took to help them get from one Power Burn meal to another.

Bouillon can double your weight loss. As part of a Pennsylvania State University study, 200 overweight and obese women ate either 1 or 2 servings of low-calorie soup; 2 servings of energy-dense, high-calorie snack foods; or no special foods. Everyone lost weight—but after 1 year, the group who had 2 daily servings of low-calorie soup lost 50 percent more weight than those who ate the same number of calories as high-calorie snack foods. The researchers believe the full bellies of the soup group really gave them the edge.[43]

The Beverages of the 2 Day Diabetes Diet

On this plan, you'll sip plenty of water as well as 2 daily servings of reduced-fat 2% milk (or yogurt). It's okay to enjoy seltzer, coffee, and hot or iced tea (either unsweetened or with a no-calorie sweetener), too. Here's what you need to know about the science behind 2 Day Diabetes Diet drinks:

Water: A tall glass of water or seltzer can help reduce dehydration and fill you up, especially if you drink it just before or with a meal. Drink your water however you like it: hot, cold, or room temperature. Jazz it up with a squeeze of lemon or lime, but don't add extra calories by flavoring it with juice.

> Jazz up your water with a squeeze of lemon or lime.

Milk: As we mentioned earlier, milk provides healthy fats, calcium, magnesium, potassium, and vitamin D and other nutrients that are good for your overall health. On the 2 Day Diabetes Diet, you'll choose 2% milk or a milk substitute (see "I'm Lactose Intolerant. Can I Still Follow This Plan?" on page 84 for more on milk substitutes).

Coffee: Some research suggests that coffee drinkers are at lower risk for developing diabetes, while other studies performed on people who already have diabetes suggest coffee may raise blood sugar or prompt the body to work harder to absorb it.[44] Should you skip or sip coffee? If you're having difficulty controlling your blood sugar, it may be worth cutting back on coffee to see if it makes a difference. Otherwise, a few cups a day are fine. If you use milk in your coffee, make sure to count that as part of your dairy allotment for the day. Don't, however, add sugar.

Tea: Black, green, and white tea contain antioxidants that may have blood sugar benefits. The bonus: no calories (provided you skip sugar, as we recommend). Sipping four cups of tea a day lowered risk for developing diabetes by 2 percent in one 2012 study by a German research group called The InterAct Consortium.[45] So sip tea as you wish—just be careful about enjoying caffeinated types close to bedtime. Herbal teas are another delicious, calorie-free option, and some, such as cinnamon tea, can

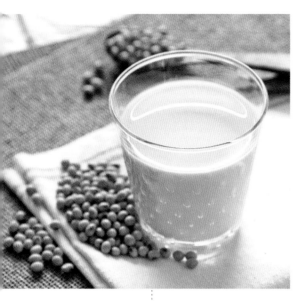

help you get blood sugar under control. Again, if you use milk, make sure to count that as part of your dairy allotment for the day.

What won't you be drinking on the 2 Day Diabetes Diet? We'd like you to avoid high-calorie, high-sugar beverage traps like soft drinks, sweet juices, sweetened iced tea, milk shakes, and specialty coffee drinks. These can elevate blood sugar and slow weight loss. We'd also like you to limit diet drinks, as some research suggests that diet soda drinkers are 6 percent more likely to develop diabetes and more likely to gain weight, too.[46] Experts suspect that one reason diet soda leads to weight gain and diabetes is that we don't usually pair zero-calorie drinks with healthy fare. The artificial sweetness of these beverages may cause us to crave sweet flavors even more, causing us to eat more cookies, cake, and other treats.[47]

If you just have to have a soda, choosing a zero-calorie version over a sugary one once or twice a week is okay. Alcohol is also allowed on the 2 Day Diabetes Diet: In fact, a serving of wine, beer, or even liquor can be used as one of your two weekly treats. Alcohol is, however, rich in calories, so drinking too much can significantly slow your weight-loss progress.

Now that you've learned all about what these individual foods can do, let's put them all together and get to work. It's time to learn the rules of the 2 Day Diabetes Diet. In just a few short pages, you'll be well on your way to seeing big results!

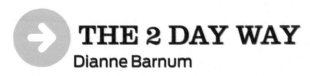

THE 2 DAY WAY
Dianne Barnum

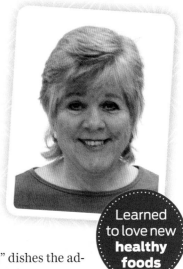

Learned to love new **healthy foods**

Dianne Barnum, 61, saw her doctor on a Tuesday and found that she had a blood glucose reading of 119 mg/dl (6.6 mmol/l). "He said, 'The next time you come to see me, unless this number is under 100, you'll be looking at starting medication.' It was a real wake-up call—one that compelled me to try the 2 Day Diabetes Diet. I'm so grateful I did."

Still, Dianne had never eaten a bean before joining the 2 Day Diabetes Diet. "Don't believe me? Oh, but it gets worse!" dishes the administrative assistant from Brookfield, Connecticut. "I'd never eaten a sweet potato, kale, collard green, or even cinnamon—unless it was embedded in a thick slab of apple pie! How the heck did I manage that?"

That was then, however—now, post–2 Day trial: "I had sweet potato fries on the diet and loved them," says Dianne. "Let me emphasize that: I. Am. In. Love. I probably have sweet potatoes twice a week now. I don't put any butter on them, maybe just a little cinnamon [because] it's good for your blood sugar."

During her six weeks on the 2 Day Diabetes Diet, Dianne dropped from a size 20 to a size 16. "Needless to say, I'm planning to stay on the diet or a variation of it forever," she says. "It just works."

The key to the 2 Day, Dianne's way:

▶ **She pushed through her mental blocks concerning Power Burn Days.** "At first I thought I was starving those days," says Dianne, "but it was 100 percent psychosomatic."

▶ **She didn't balk at the initial bump in her grocery bill.** "When you have to buy almond butter for the first time, for instance, your grocery bill is going to go up," Dianne says. "But these products tend to last forever."

▶ **She tried a few on-the-plate tricks.** "I used to eat my salad with my meal," says Dianne. "Now, I begin every meal with a salad and I eat less during dinner. I also plate the food in my kitchen; keeping it out of sight has helped me to curb my urge to have more and more and more, even after I'm full."

CHAPTER 5

How to Follow the 2 Day Diabetes Diet

Three levels make this diet flexible, inclusive, and easy to personalize to your tastes, your lifestyle, and your personality.

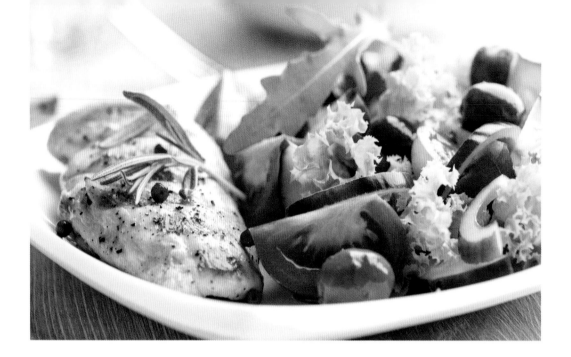

We've supplied you with a lot of information so far. If you feel a little overwhelmed—as if you couldn't possibly remember it all—we've got one word for you: relax. We've got you covered. This chapter serves as an at-a-glance resource, one that houses everything you need to know about following the 2 Day Diabetes Diet in an easy-to-digest format. Skim over it now, and refer to it as needed.

Getting started on the 2 Day Diabetes Diet is as simple as 3 easy steps, all of which you can accomplish in the next 5 minutes, without even getting out of your chair.

Step 1: Pick the Right Level for You

The 2 Day Diabetes Diet includes three levels that differ not in food composition or calories, but in flexibility.

> ▶ **Level 1** provides specific menus for every day. If you are the kind of a dieter who loves structure and who hates ambiguity, this is the perfect place to start. You'll find the Level 1 eating plan in Chapter 6.

- **Level 2** provides mix and match menus. To follow this level, all you need to do is choose from the dozens of breakfast, lunch, dinner, and snack options. We've done all the number crunching for you. You'll find the Level 2 eating plan in Chapter 7.
- **Level 3** provides the most flexibility, and we recommend you don't start this level until you've gotten used to the diet by spending several weeks in Level 1 or 2. In Level 3, you will find an easy-to-use formula that allows you to create your own 2 Day Diabetes Diet Power Burn and Nourishment meals. You'll find the Level 3 formulas in Chapter 8.

Step 2: Decide When to Power Burn

No matter which level of the plan you follow, you will power burn 2 days a week and nourish the other 5. It's important to pick your Power Burn Days before you start. Otherwise, you run the risk of telling yourself, "I'll power burn tomorrow." Then tomorrow comes and you might tell yourself, "No, today is too busy. I'll try it tomorrow."

Then tomorrow never comes.

So take a moment now and think about which days might work best for power burning and which for nourishing. You'll want to do this even if you plan to start with Level 1. Yes, we've worked the Power Burn Days into your Level 1 plan, but you still have some flexibility. You can rearrange the Level 1 eating schedule as needed.

Are you like many dieters who prefer to power burn on the weekends when you can take things easy and not worry about toting special foods to work? Or do you prefer to do it during the workweek when your job will help to distract you from the fact that you are dieting? Do some days, just by the nature of your schedule, work better for power burning than other days? You can make any 2 days of the week your Power Burn Days; it doesn't matter if you space them out or schedule them back to back. Whatever works for you is the best way. Just don't do 3 Power Burn Days

FAQ: I'M WORRIED MY BLOOD SUGAR WILL DROP. WHAT SHOULD I KNOW AND DO?

Our test panelists experienced no instances of hypoglycemia, even those on insulin! However, we understand this is a real concern. If you are prone to low blood sugar, follow this advice.

▶ Test your blood sugar at least 3 times a day: after fasting, 2 hours after eating, and before bed. If you exercise, make sure to test both before and after exercise and plan to eat before and after a workout to prevent drops in blood sugar.

▶ If your sugar tests low (below 70 mg/dl or 3.9 mmol/l), use the 15/15 Rule to correct a low blood sugar episode. Eat 15 grams of carbs, wait 15 minutes, and retest. Repeat until your blood sugar is within the normal range (80–100 mg/dl 4.4 -5.5 mmol/l).

▶ On both Nourishment and Power Burn Days, stay within the total portion recommendations per day, but consider splitting up your meals so you are eating more frequently. Divide the meals or snacks into smaller amounts so you can eat six small meals/snacks per day to prevent hypoglycemia.

▶ Plan exercise accordingly as well; you may want to reserve it for Nourishment Days and be less active on Power Burn Days. Plan to eat a source of carbohydrate both before and after exercise or any physical activity to prevent drops in blood sugar.

in a row (for instance, 2 at the end of one week, and 1 at the beginning of the next). This will be too stressful on your body.

Even though we are suggesting you pick power burning days now, this doesn't mean you must power burn on the same days from week to week. If, for example, you usually have a Power Burn Day on Thursdays, but this week you'll be at a dinner party, you can make Thursday a Nourishment Day to allow for some extra calories. (You still have to eat healthy on Nourishment Days, of course.) It is, however, helpful to start each week with a sense of which days you will Power Burn and which ones you will set aside for Nourishment.

Here are some additional pointers.

▷ If the idea of power burning seems too hard, you may want to start by scheduling one or more Nourishment Days in between your Power Days. This will provide a break between your dieting days, much as taking a nap in the midafternoon can help you sustain a long study session that flows into the evening hours.

▷ At least in the beginning, exercise only on Nourishment Days. On Power Burn Days, exercise lightly or not at all. After you've been on the plan for a while, you'll develop a sense of how much exercise you can handle on a Power Burn Day; depending on your fitness level, you may not find a difference.

- We highly recommend you do Tension Tamers on Power Burn Days. You'll find a list of them in Chapter 10. Tension Tamers are incredibly useful during those moments when you are faced with hunger or a craving.
- Save treats for Nourishment Days. You can choose two treats per week, but don't indulge on Power Burn Days.

Step 3: Decide When to Snack

No matter what level of the plan you are following, you'll consume one snack a day at the time of day that works best for you. A good rule of thumb is to consume your snack during the longest stretch of time between meals. So if you usually tend to have 3 hours between breakfast and lunch but 6 hours between lunch and dinner, you'll probably want to plan to have your snack between lunch and dinner.

We also encourage you to add in two weekly treats. We've worked these treats into your Level 1 plan. In Levels 2 and 3, you'll find a treat list from which to choose. Incorporate those treats on Nourishment Days.

Additional Pointers

For best results, use the following advice no matter which level of the plan you are following.

Consume recommended beverages only. Make water your mainstay, and aim for at least eight 8-ounce glasses a day. Turn to it especially on Power Burn Days. Down a glass of water before meals and also whenever you feel hungry. Many of our panelists found that downing a glass of water helped to turn down hunger during Power Burn Days. Other recommended beverages include 2% milk, tea, and coffee. Ideally you'll consume water, reduced-fat milk, tea, or coffee only. But if you just have to have a soda, choosing a zero-calorie version over a sugary one once or twice a week is okay. Omit other beverages such as fruit and vegetable juices.

Space out your meals as evenly as possible. This helps keep your blood sugar levels steady and your appetite under control. On Power Burn Days, when you eat less than other times of the week, this is a particularly helpful tactic. Most of us don't have total control over our daily mealtimes, so don't stress over your eating schedule too much. But to the extent that you can avoid it don't, for example, eat lunch just an hour or two after breakfast, leaving a long stretch before dinner.

Exercise on Nourishment Days. Exercise is optional but recommended. It will help you get results even faster. Plus, the research is very clear: Activity is not only key to helping you maintain a healthy weight, but it can also help even out your blood sugar levels. So we strongly recommend it. If you already have a regular exercise routine that's working for you, by all means stick to it! If you are not already exercising, start when you feel ready. As you lose weight on the 2 Day Diabetes Diet and your blood sugar levels normalize, you'll have more energy, making exercise easier. For inspiration and guidance, use the routines in Chapter 11. Our exercise plan includes three types of movement: walking, strength-training, and tummy-flattening moves. Here's how you'll work those routines into your eating schedule.

Walking: Do your walking at least three times a week, on Nourishment Days.

Strength training: Do our nine-move routine twice a week, leaving one to two rest days in between for optimal muscle recovery. The full routine takes about 20 minutes, but feel free to break it up into three 6- to 7-minute sequences focused on your upper body, your core, and your lower body (we'll show you how) that you can do at different times of day or even on different days. You can add more repetitions of each exercise as your strength increases.

Tummy flattening: Do these moves in conjunction with your strength-training routine.

> Switch back and forth among the different levels of the plan as often as you'd like.

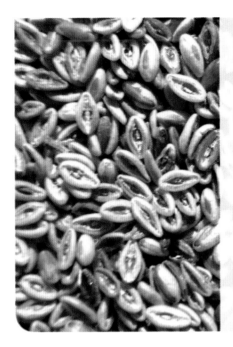

SUPERFOOD SPOTLIGHT:
Psyllium Husk

Why do the delicious, homemade fruit smoothies on the 2 Day Diabetes Diet contain a teaspoon of ground psyllium along with tasty ingredients like yogurt, vanilla extract, cherries, apples, blueberries, and mangoes? This add-in, long used for constipation relief, is proven to help people with diabetes control blood sugar better. A 2010 review from the University of California, San Diego, published in the *Annals of Pharmacotherapy,* confirms this benefit .[1] People who took psyllium before a meal saw their post-meal blood sugar levels rise 2 percent less than those who didn't use this supplement.[2] One caution: The researchers recommend waiting at least 4 hours after taking psyllium before taking medications because psyllium can decrease their absorption.

Tame tension on Power Burn Days. Do the relaxation exercises twice a week, on Power Burn Days. Choose your favorite relaxation exercises from the ones listed in Chapter 10. Research shows that cultivating calm also gives your weight-loss and blood sugar–control efforts a powerful boost. Choose the Belly-Breathing Exercise or the Sighing Exercise (it also uses breath to relax you) when you've got just a few minutes, and the Muscle Relaxation Technique or Limb Relaxation Exercise when you've got about 10 minutes.

Follow the plan as long as needed. Feel free to switch back and forth among the different levels of the plan as often as you'd like, but try to stay on the plan until you reach the results you want. You might see results in as few as 3 weeks (as our test panelists did), but we recommend you stick with the 2 Day Diabetes Diet for at least 6, as this is long enough to see lasting changes in blood sugar. Ideally you'll stay on it until you've dropped all the pounds you want and have your blood sugar numbers under control. When that happens, use the advice in Chapter 12 to maintain those results for life.

THE 2 DAY WAY
Karen Lerch

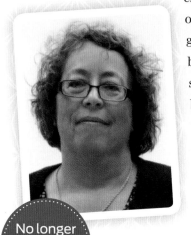

No longer **at risk** for diabetes

Not surprisingly, Karen Lerch, a British expat with a daisy chain of diet failures behind her, adores European chocolate. "You know those delicious chocolate bunnies?" she asks. "I cannot tell you how many of those I've bought over the years for my children only to gobble them up myself! No wonder I'd gotten myself in trouble. I came very close to being diagnosed with diabetes," she says. When she started the 2 Day Diabetes Diet, her fasting blood sugar was 108 mg/dl (6 mmol/l), firmly in prediabetes territory.

She also weighed 183 pounds and had already tried many diets. Karen had tried Weight Watchers. She'd tried South Beach. And yet the 52-year-old German teacher in Mount Arlington, New Jersey, found herself facing menopause and life post-divorce grossly overweight, taking medication for both high blood pressure and high cholesterol, with the specter of a diabetes diagnosis looming. "I had no man and no money; my modus operandi was to turn to comfort foods to make myself feel better," she says. "So I knew, going in to the 2 Day Diet, that if I was going to lose weight, I had to feel satisfied emotionally—and, on this diet, I do."

The 2 Day Diabetes Diet, proved to be a way of eating this self-described all-occasion-eater ("Even when I'm sick, I eat," she groans) could stick with. And that's a monumental first for her.

The proof is in the numbers: After just 6 weeks on the 2 Day Diabetes Diet, Karen dropped 8 pounds and a whopping 4 ½ inches from her waist. Her fasting blood sugar also dropped 32 points—that's a 30 percent decrease! Now it's 76 mg/dl (4.2 mmol/L), and she is no longer considered at risk for diabetes.

"I now have a sense that a waist is out there somewhere, just waiting for me" she pealed. "I'm doing the disappearing act, my own little vanishing act. And I love it. I'm very pleased."

The key to the 2 Day, Karen's way:

- ▶ **She checked in on her body chemistry often.** "Just realizing that I could test my blood sugar level at will was very, very motivating for me," says Karen. "It was another tool to measure my progress, and as I think most women can agree, it's just really nice sometimes to have something other than the scale to grade you."

- ▶ **She resisted carbs.** "It actually wasn't all that hard," says Karen. "They were my nemesis before, but after being on the diet for several weeks, I no longer craved them. It helps that I'm a soup girl. I really like the broth—I often put spinach in it—so I'm not even hungry on Power Burn Days. Honestly, I'm not hungry on any days of the diet, and that has never happened with me."

- ▶ **She didn't give up.** "Remember, slow and sure wins the race," says Karen. "I'd love to morph into some skinny Minnie overnight, and before trying the 2 Day Diabetes Diet, I would get discouraged if I didn't lose a bunch of weight quickly. But I like my progress on the 2 Day and, more importantly, I like how I feel. I could feel that the diet was working right away. And even now that I can see that the diet is working, I'm not feeling deprived. What I'm feeling is happy. Really, *really* happy."

CHAPTER 6

Level 1: The 2 Week Quick Start Plan

A two-week day-by-day starter menu makes weight loss simple. Just shop, chop, and watch the fat melt away and your blood sugar levels stabilize.

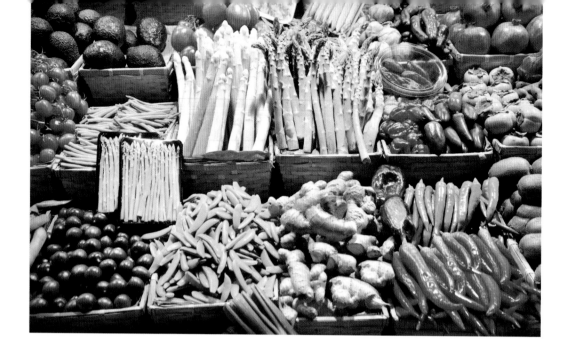

We've given you the science. We've told you about the foods. You have the guidelines.

Ready to dig in?

In this chapter, you'll find a 2 week starter menu to show you what your 2 Day Diabetes Diet looks like. Level 1 is a great place to start the diet, especially if you are the kind of person who loves structure. If you follow the menus exactly as presented, all the decisions and work have been done for you. We've even written your shopping list.

Level 1 also will give your brain the practice it needs to turn this new way of eating into a habit—and you'll be on your way that much faster to a leaner waist, a stronger heart, and a lifetime of vibrant, diabetes-free health. It's time to sink your teeth into a perfectly broiled pork tenderloin and some satisfying Baked Sweet Potato "Fries" (page 238). It's your turn to spoon up some Carrot Soup with Dill (page 185) or sip a sweet Black Cherry Smoothie (page 251), too. Most important: It's time to get your blood sugar under control and nudge those numbers on the scale downward.

FORGIVENESS IS A VIRTUE—AND A SUCCESS TOOL

Maybe you got tempted by the jar of jelly beans on a coworker's desk. Maybe you ended up going out to dinner, and the desserts were sooooo tempting. It's okay! Mistakes are inevitable in any venture. Whatever went wrong, it's not worth getting upset and stressed over, and it's certainly no cause to give up. Just move forward and stick to the next day's schedule.

No Menu Planning Required

The beauty of this method: You don't have to plan anything. Erin has done all the work for you. She's even assembled shopping lists for you. If you simply incorporate the choices in the order she suggests, there's no thinking required.

That said, you have some wiggle room. These meal plans are meant as a guideline, not gospel. If you're allergic to a specific ingredient, or you just plain don't like the taste of something, then you can easily switch that dish for another meal—feel free to pick and choose from the meal options you'll find later in this chapter. The only caveat is that you must pick an equivalent: For example, you can swap a Power Burn breakfast for another Power Burn breakfast, or a Nourishment dinner for another Nourishment dinner. You can even swap a Nourishment lunch for a Nourishment dinner and vice versa. Just don't do the same on Power Burn Days, as Power Burn lunches and dinners contain differing numbers of calories.

As far as shuffling the meals within the days themselves, though, go nuts! If on Day 1 you wanted to have your wrap first thing in the morning, the Summer Garden Soup (page 186) for lunch, and Banana Toast (page 174) for dinner, that would be fine.

Also, you can swap whole days. So if you don't want to do your Power Burn Day on Day 3, as written, you can simply eat Day 4's meals on Day 3 and Day 3's meals on Day 4.

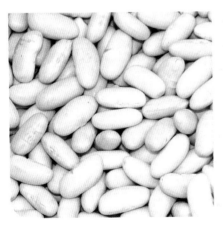

SUPERFOOD SPOTLIGHT:
Cannellini Beans

Packed with protein and cholesterol-lowering soluble fiber, legumes such as tender, white cannellini beans are slow to raise blood sugar. As part of a 2012 University of Toronto study, 121 people with type 2 diabetes followed a healthy diet containing a daily cup of beans or whole grains. After 3 months, the bean group saw their A1c levels—a check of average blood sugar levels—fall nearly twice as much as the whole-grain group.[1]

Your Prep Work

For most people, the hardest part of a diet is the beginning—and especially the very first week. That's when everything feels new and perhaps a bit foreign. During this week you might be cooking recipes you've never before tried and even shopping for ingredients you've never before purchased.

It will all go more smoothly, however, if you do a little prep work. For optimal success, do the following before you dig in.

▶ Take a look at the menu options and the accompanying recipes. Decide whether you will need some swaps or follow the plan as is. Make any necessary adjustments to the Week 1 shopping list on page 105.

▶ Using the shopping list as a guide, check your kitchen cabinets. Note what you have on hand and what you do not. Head to the grocery store and stock up.

▶ Unless otherwise noted, you should eat 1 serving of a recipe per meal. (Recipes are provided in Chapter 9.) Note that we want you to use 2% milk and low-fat yogurt. In general, this should be plain yogurt but flavored yogurts are okay if artificially sweetened. Added sugar in yogurt is a no-no.

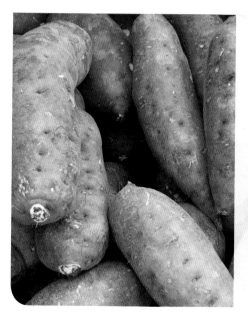

SUPERFOOD SPOTLIGHT:
Sweet Potatoes

Sweet potatoes provide an astonishing variety of nutritional benefits. One analysis found that sweet potatoes reduce HgbA1c measures between 0.30 and 0.57 percent and fasting blood glucose by 10 to 15 points.[2] Sweet potato also contains anthocyanins, the natural pigments that give the sweet potato its deep orange color.[3] Anthocyanins are the Swiss army knife of antioxidants, believed to have anti-inflammatory, antiviral, and antimicrobial qualities. Sweet potatoes have such a deeply satisfying creamy sweetness—they don't need any maple syrup or marshmallows! Keep it simple—simply pierce a sweet potato and throw it in the oven at 375 degrees for an hour.

Your Week 1 Shopping List

Use this checklist to see what you already have on hand as well as what you must purchase so you're prepared for each week of the 2 Week Quick Start Plan.

Week 1 Essentials

Produce

Apple, 1 medium

Arugula, 1 ½ cups

Asparagus spears, 1 ½ pounds

Bananas, 2

Basil leaves, fresh

Bell peppers, green, 2 medium

Bell peppers, red, 3 medium

Blackberries, fresh or frozen, 2 cups

Blueberries, 2 cups

Broccoli, fresh or frozen, 1 cup

Carrots, raw, 2 pounds

Celery, fresh, 2 stalks

Collard greens, fresh or frozen, ½ cup

Cucumber, 1

Dates, 6

Flat-leaf parsley, 1 cup

Garlic, 11 cloves

Ginger, fresh, 1 piece

Grapes, purple or green, 1 cup

Green beans, fresh or frozen, ¼ pound

Green peas, fresh or frozen, 1 ¾ cups

Hot peppers, 4

Leeks, 2

Lemon, 1

Mint, fresh, ⅔ cup

Mushrooms, 2 cups

Olives, pitted ripe, 10 medium

Onions, 10 medium

Orange, 1 medium

Peach, 1 medium

Radishes, 4

Raisins, 5 tablespoons

Red onions, 3 medium

Red potatoes, 1 pound

Russet potatoes, 2 medium

Salad in a bag or fresh lettuce

Spinach, fresh, 4 cups

Spinach, frozen, chopped, 2 packages (10 ounces each)

Sweet potatoes, 2

Thyme leaves, fresh, ¼ cup

Tomatoes, 4 fresh

Tomatoes, plum, 6

Yellow summer squash, 1 medium

Zucchini, 1 medium

Miscellaneous Packaged Foods

Almond butter, natural

Applesauce, unsweetened, ½ cup

Beef bouillon cube, 1

Broth, chicken or vegetable, 28 ounces

Cereal, 100% whole grain

Dark chocolate, 70% cacao or higher, 1 ounce

Hummus, 1 small container

Lemon juice

Peanut butter, natural

Peanuts, raw or dry roasted, ¼ cup

popchips, baked, 1-ounce bag

Tomato paste, 1 can (4 ounces)

Tomato sauce or pizza sauce, 1 cup

Tomatoes, crushed, 1 can (28 ounces)

Tomatoes, diced, 2 cans (14 ½ ounces each)

Walnuts, raw or dry roasted, ½ cup

Wooden skewers, 3

Grains

Bulgur, 2 cups

Flour, all-purpose, ½ cup

Pasta, 100% whole grain, 2 ounces

Wild rice

Condiments

Artificial sweetener, if desired

Hot red-pepper sauce, 1 tablespoon

Roasted red pepper

Worcestershire sauce

Spices

Bay leaf, 1

Cinnamon

Curry powder

Dill, 1 tablespoon

Fennel seeds, crushed (can substitute dried oregano instead)

Garlic powder

Garlic salt

Onion powder

Oregano

Paprika

Rosemary, fresh or dried

Salt, iodized

Thyme, dried, ½ teaspoon

Vanilla extract, 1 tablespoon

White pepper

Meat and Fish

Beef, ground,
   93% lean,
   1 pound

Canadian bacon,
   1 ounce

Chicken breasts,
   skinless,
   3 pounds

Cod, scrod,
   halibut, or other
   thick, firm-
   fleshed white
   fish steaks,
   1 pound

Flank steak,
   5 ounces

Flounder, fresh,
   5 ounces

Pork tenderloin,
   5 ounces

Shrimp, fresh
   or frozen
   uncooked,
   peeled and
   deveined,
   2 pounds

Turkey breast
   meat, ground,
   13 ounces

Turkey breast,
   low-sodium deli
   meat, sliced,
   5 ounces

Eggs and Dairy

Egg whites, liquid

Eggs

Gruyère or
   Jarlsberg cheese,
   shredded, about
   2 tablespoons

Margarine spread,
   trans fat free

Milk, 2%, 8 cups

Parmesan
   cheese, low
   fat, grated

Mozzarella
   cheese, reduced
   fat, shredded,
   about 1 ½ cups

Ricotta cheese,
   part skim,
   ½ cup

Yogurt, plain 2%,
   10 cups

Bread

Arnold's
   Sandwich Thins

Bread crumbs,
   fresh, ½ cup

Bread, 100%
   whole grain

Breadstick, whole
   grain, 1

Pitas, 100%
   whole grain
   (4" diameter), 5

Tortillas, 100%
   whole grain
   (6" diameter), 2

Oils

Canola oil

Nonstick cooking
   spray

Olive oil

Vegetable oil (can
   replace
   with canola oil)

Vinaigrette salad
   dressing,
   5 grams or less
   of sugar per
   serving

Frozen Foods

Waffles, frozen, 100% whole grain, 2

Two Weeks to a Slimmer, Healthier You

You'll find 2 weeks' worth of menus in the following pages. When preparing meals, it's important to stick to the measurements and serving sizes we've given you, especially on Power Burn Days, so you don't undermine the progress you're making. That being said, don't go crazy measuring everything exactly; a fraction of a teaspoon here or an extra calorie there is not going to make that big of a difference in the long run. Note that some of our recipes yield multiple servings, so save some for another day! In a few cases, your meal option gives you 2 servings (or sometimes ½ a serving) of a recipe, so read carefully when planning your meals. Remember that you can move your Power Burn Days around to wherever suits you during the week.

Week 1

	BREAKFAST	LUNCH	DINNER	SNACK
Day 1	Banana Toast **(page 174)**, 1 c low-fat yogurt	Wrap made with one 12" whole-grain tortilla, rolled with 5 oz deli turkey breast, ½ c sliced raw hot peppers, ¼ c sliced onion, ¼ c diced tomato, and 2 Tbsp hummus, served with 1 c garden salad and 1 Tbsp dressing on the side	1 serving **Summer Garden Soup (page 186)**, served with 5 oz broiled pork tenderloin, 3 oz sweet potato topped with 1 tsp trans-fat-free spread, and ½ c prepared collard greens sautéed in 1 tsp olive oil	Sliced apple topped with cinnamon, 1 c 2% milk
	BREAKFAST	**LUNCH**	**DINNER**	**SNACK**
Day 2	Yogurt parfait made with 1 c low-fat yogurt, layered with ½ c whole-grain cereal and 1 c blackberries, topped with 1 Tbsp chopped walnuts	5 oz turkey breast grilled and served on 1 Arnold's Sandwich Thin and 1 serving **Baked Sweet Potato "Fries" (page 238)** with 2 c salad greens and 1 Tbsp vinaigrette dressing	2 servings **Tabbouleh (page 243)** served with 5 oz broiled flounder	**Black Cherry Smoothie (page 251)**

	BREAKFAST	LUNCH	DINNER	SNACK	
Day 3 **Power Burn Day**	Omelet made with 2 egg whites and ½ c onions and peppers cooked in nonfat cooking spray, 1 c low-fat yogurt	1 serving **Carrot Soup with Dill (page 185)**, served with 1 c fresh blueberries	½ serving **Spinach-Stuffed Meat Loaf (page 199)**, served with ½ c steamed broccoli, 1 c 2% milk	1 c purple or green grapes	

	BREAKFAST	LUNCH	DINNER	SNACK	TREAT
Day 4	1 whole-grain waffle topped with 1 c berries and 1 c low-fat yogurt topped with 1 Tbsp chopped walnuts	6" pita stuffed with 4 oz grilled chicken breast, 2 Tbsp hummus, and ½ c roasted red peppers, served with **Baked Tomato (page 240)**	1 serving **Baked Cod Casserole with Potatoes, Tomatoes, and Arugula (page 214)**, with 1 serving **Tex-Mex Red Beans (page 244)**	1 c low-fat yogurt topped with 3 dates and 1 tsp ground cinnamon	1 oz baked popchips

	BREAKFAST	LUNCH	DINNER	SNACK	
Day 5 **Power Burn Day**	1 oz Canadian bacon, ½ c frozen spinach, cooked, 1 c 2% milk	**Bouillon Vegetable Soup (page 183)**, ½ banana topped with 2 tsp peanut butter	**Grilled Chicken Kabobs (page 204)**, ½ c zucchini cooked with cooking spray over ¼ c whole-grain pasta, 1 c 2% milk	1 medium orange	

	BREAKFAST	LUNCH	DINNER	SNACK	TREAT
Day 6	½ c whole-grain cereal with ½ c 2% milk and ½ c low-fat yogurt layered with 3 dates and 1 Tbsp chopped peanuts	2 servings **Pita Pizza (page 223)**, and 1 c garden salad topped with 4 oz grilled, sliced chicken breast and 2 Tbsp vinaigrette, 1 small breadstick	1 serving **Curried Chicken Dinner (page 205)**, served with 1 serving **Bulgur with Spring Vegetables (page 242)**	**Yogurt Fruit Dip (page 248)**, 1 peach cut into slices and dipped	1 oz dark chocolate

	BREAKFAST	LUNCH	DINNER	SNACK	
Day 7	**Peanut Butter Tortilla (page 174)**, 1 c low-fat yogurt	¾ c **Zippy Shrimp (page 218)**, served over 2 c fresh spinach leaves topped with 2 Tbsp vinaigrette and 1 c prepared wild rice	5 oz flank steak, broiled, topped with 1 c mushrooms/onions sautéed in 1 tsp olive oil, and 3 oz sweet potato with 1 tsp trans-fat-free spread	**Apple-Cinnamon Smoothie (page 250)**	

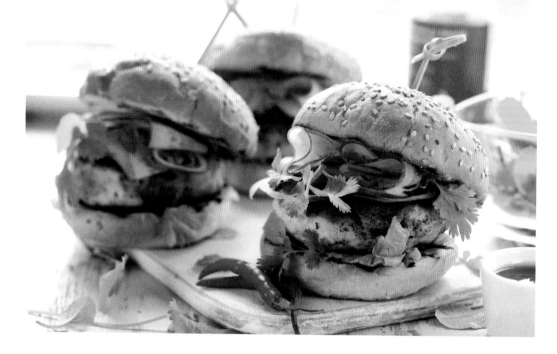

Ready for Week Two?

Have you already experienced some success and dropped a pound or two on the scale? If so, congrats!

If not, examine why that might be. Did you stick to the menus closely? Did you make substitutions? Did you do the Power Burn days? Be honest but also be kind to yourself. This isn't about feeling guilty. It's about solving problems and overcoming obstacles to your success. Maybe you want to try power burning on different days of the week. Or maybe you want to line up more support from friends or family. It's also quite possible that patience is all you need. Sometimes our bodies just need a period of adjustment before they are ready to drop pounds. You might be pleasantly surprised next week when you step on the scale!

Before you start Week 2, take a look at the following shopping list. Check your cabinets to see what you already have on hand and what you don't. Many of the shopping items are carryovers from Week 1, so you should be set. If you are missing anything, head to the store to stock up.

Then look over the menus for the weeks to come. As with Week 1, feel free to shuffle some meals around to suit your tastes and lifestyle, perhaps moving a Power Burn Day earlier or later in the week, for instance. Enjoy!

Week 2 Essentials

Produce

Apples, 2 medium

Bell peppers, red, 2 medium

Bell pepper, yellow, 1 medium

Bell peppers, green, 3 medium

Berries, any variety, 1 cup

Blueberries, fresh or frozen, 1 cup

Bok choy, small, or other Chinese greens, ½ pound

Broccoli, 1 pound raw

Carrots, raw, 1 ½ pounds

Cauliflower, ½ cup

Celery, 6 large stalks

Cherries, tart, dried, 2

Collard greens, 2 small bunches

Dates, 3

Garlic, 10 cloves

Ginger, fresh, 2 slices (if no leftovers from Week 1)

Honeydew melon, sliced, 1 cup

Leeks, 2

Mango, 1 cup

Mushrooms, 1 ½ cups

Onions, 7 large

Peach, 1

Pear, 1 medium

Pineapple, 1 ¼ cups

Plums, 2

Potatoes, Yukon Gold or all-purpose, 2 medium

Salad, 1 pre-made bag

Scallions, 4

Strawberries, fresh, 1 cup

Sugar snaps, ¾ cup

Swiss chard, 1 small bunch

Tomato, 1 medium

Miscellaneous Packaged Foods

Bouillon, beef or vegetable, 2 cubes

Broth, chicken, reduced sodium, fat free, 3 cans (14 ½ ounces each)

Cannellini beans, 1 cup

Cookie, 1 small

Cornstarch, 2 teaspoons

Granola, ¼ cup

Kidney beans, 1 can (16 ounces)

Kidney beans, red, dried, 1 cup

Lime juice, ⅔ cup

Pecans, chopped, 1 tablespoon

Tomatoes, crushed, 3 cans (14 ounces each)

Tomatoes, diced, ½ cup

V8 juice, 1 can (46 ounces)

Vegetable stock, 1 cup

Wine, white or sake, 2 tablespoons

Grains

Brown rice noodles, 1 cup

Couscous, whole grain, 1 ½ cups

Oats, steel cut, ½ cup

Pancake mix, 100% whole grain

Pasta, 100% whole grain, ¼ cup

Psyllium husk, 1 teaspoon

Quinoa, ⅓ cup

Condiments

Browning sauce, ⅛ teaspoon

Honey, 3 tablespoons

Mayonnaise, regular or light

Soy sauce, reduced sodium, ½ cup

Thai fish sauce, 1 tablespoon

Spices

Basil, dried

Bay leaves, 2

Celery seed

Cayenne pepper

Chili powder

Cocoa powder, 1 teaspoon

Cumin

Mustard, ground

Sugar, dark brown, 1 teaspoon

Turmeric, ground, 1 teaspoon

Meat and Fish

Beef round steak, 1 pound

Chicken breast, 7 ounces

Flank steak, 2 ounces

Halibut or other firm-fleshed white fish fillets, 1 ½ pounds

Pork loin chops (4 ounces each), 6 boneless

Pork, center chop, 5 ounces

Salmon, filet, 5 ounces

Tuna steak, 5 ounces

Turkey breast, ground, 4 ounces or pre-made 4-ounce turkey breast burger

Turkey breast, sliced, 4 ounces

Eggs and Dairy

Cheese, low fat, any variety, 2 ounces	Milk, 2%, 7 cups	Parmesan cheese block, 1 ounce	Yogurt, 2% plain, 8 cups

Bread

Bread, 100% whole grain Bread, 100% whole grain, reduced calorie, 4 slices	Egg whites, liquid (1 cup or 8 egg whites)	English muffin, 100% whole grain, 1 Hamburger bun, 100% whole grain, 1	Tortilla, 100% whole grain, one 12"

Oils

Balsamic vinegar

Frozen Foods

Ice cream, ½ cup

Week 2

	BREAKFAST	LUNCH	DINNER	SNACK
Day 1 Power Burn Day	Mushroom Quiche (page 113), topped with ½ c diced tomatoes and 1 c 2% milk	1 serving **Warm Green Vegetable Salad with Garlic and Ginger (page 191),** served with 8 oz prepared bouillon and 1 c 2% plain yogurt topped with 1 c fresh strawberries	2 servings **Roasted Carrots with Rosemary (page 237)** with 2 oz broiled flank steak served on 1 slice of reduced-calorie bread and 1 c 2% milk	2 small plums
	BREAKFAST	LUNCH	DINNER	SNACK
Day 2	Baked Apple (page 179), 1 c low-fat yogurt topped with ¼ c granola	1 serving **Round Steak Chili (page 180),** served with 3 slices reduced-calorie light bread, topped with 2 tsp trans-fat-free spread, 1 tsp garlic powder, and 4 Tbsp Parmesan cheese (spread evenly over each slice of bread and toast until melted)	2 servings **Creamy Greens Soup (page 188),** served with 5 oz grilled tuna steak, ½ c steamed broccoli, and ⅓ c cooked quinoa	Blueberry Smoothie (page 252)
	BREAKFAST	LUNCH	DINNER	SNACK
Day 3	½ whole-grain English muffin topped with 2 tsp nut butter, ½ c pineapple, and 1 c 2% milk	5 oz sautéed chicken breast in 2 tsp olive oil with garlic, 1 c prepared cannellini beans, and 1 c steamed broccoli	2 servings **Roasted Asparagus and Red Pepper with Parmesan (page 234),** served with 5 oz pork center-cut chop, ⅔ c couscous	Parfait made with alternating layers of low-fat yogurt and sliced honeydew melon
	BREAKFAST	LUNCH	DINNER	SNACK
Day 4 Power Burn Day	Baked Tomato (page 240), 1 c 2% milk	2 large celery stalks topped with 2 tsp natural nut butter, 1 serving fresh berries, 1 cup bouillon (any flavor)	Two servings **Warm Green Vegetable Salad with Garlic and Ginger (see page 191)** served with 2 oz grilled chicken, ¼ c prepared whole wheat pasta, and 1 cup 2% milk	¾ c pineapple

	BREAKFAST	LUNCH	DINNER	SNACK	TREAT
Day 5	½ c steel cut oats topped with 1 Tbs chopped pecans, cinnamon, and sliced apple, 1 c 2% milk	4 oz sliced turkey breast, 1 oz low-fat cheese on 2 slices whole-grain bread, and 1 tsp mayo (or 1 Tbsp light mayo), on 2 slices whole-grain 2 c garden salad with 2 Tbsp light vinaigrette dressing	5 oz salmon filet, grilled and served with ⅔ c whole grain couscous and 1 c cooked collard greens sautéed in 2 tsp olive oil	**Cherry Turmeric Yogurt (page 249)**	½ c ice cream

	BREAKFAST	LUNCH	DINNER	SNACK	TREAT
Day 6	½ c whole-grain cereal with ½ c 2% milk, ½ c low-fat yogurt layered with 3 dates and 1 Tbsp chopped peanuts	4 oz grilled turkey burger on whole-grain bun topped with 1 oz low-fat/fat-free cheese, served with 2 c garden salad with 2 Tbsp dressing	1 serving **Honey-Lime Pork Chops (page 203)**, served with 1 serving **Tex-Mex Red Beans (page 244)**, ½ c steamed cauliflower, and 1 slice reduced-calorie light bread with 1 tsp trans-fat-free spread	1 c lowfat yogurt topped with 1 tsp cocoa powder, 1 pear	1 small cookie

	BREAKFAST	LUNCH	DINNER	SNACK
Day 7	1 whole grain pancake topped with 1 tsp trans fat free margarine, 1 peach, 1 c 2% milk	12" whole grain tortilla topped with 5 oz low fat mozzarella cheese, ½ c tomato sauce, ½ c sautéed mushrooms and onions (cooked in 2 tsp olive oil)	1 serving **Asian Steamed Fish Fillets with Vegetable Sticks (page 217)** served with 1 cup prepared brown rice noodles tossed with 1 tsp olive oil and ½ cup prepared red peppers and onions (sautéed in 1 tsp olive oil)	**Mango Smoothie (page 252)**

Congrats!

We hope you loved every bite of Level 1. Now that you've completed 2 weeks, you've got some choices.

> **Stay in Level 1:** If you loved the 2 Week Quick Start Plan, you can go back and repeat it over and over until you reach your goal.
> **Proceed to Level 2:** If you'd like more variety and flexibility, progress to the Level 2 Mix and Match Plan in Chapter 7. This Mix and Match Plan includes dozens of options and frozen dinner suggestions, too.
> **Skip to Level 3:** If you feel confident on the plan and crave even more flexibility, progress to Level 3, found in Chapter 8. That's where you'll learn how to create your own 2 Day Diabetes Diet–friendly meals.

And after spending two weeks in the 2 Day driver's seat, now is a great time to get vocal, especially if friends and family are already asking that wonderful question, "Did you do something different with your hair? You look good."

Telling others about your efforts and your success can actually do something amazing: help you become even more successful. And you can do it in person or even online. Scientists at the University of South Carolina put 96 people on the same weight loss program but instructed half of them to use Twitter to read posts from their weight loss counselor. The participants lost an average 2.7 percent of their weight at six months, but those who also posted about their experience on Twitter lost even more. The researchers crunched the numbers and found that, for every 10 tweets a person posted about their program, they lost an additional 0.5 percent of their weight. (So if you were 200 pounds, this research suggests you might lose a pound after every 10 tweets!)[4]

So go to Twitter right now and send out a tweet. Let others know what you've been up to!

THE 2-DAY WAY
Mary Goudey

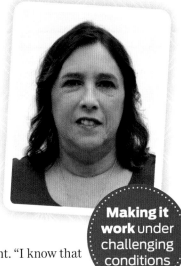

Mary Goudey comes from a long line of people with diabetes. Her mother has diabetes. Her grandmother has diabetes. Her grandfather has diabetes. And the 58-year-old hospital case manager herself has metabolic syndrome, a catchall term for a group of risk factors (such as extra weight around your middle) that occur together and increase the risk for heart disease, stroke, and—you got it—type 2 diabetes.

Making it work under challenging conditions

"I'm definitely at risk," says the Newton, New Jersey, resident. "I know that like I know my own mother. I also know that keeping my weight down, especially around my waist, is the best thing I can do to reduce that risk." This is exactly what Mary did, shaving 4 ½ inches from her waist after 6 weeks on the 2 Day Diabetes Diet—despite being battered by a certified national disaster.

Hurricane Sandy, which devastated New York and New Jersey in late October 2012, forced Mary from her home just a couple of weeks after she started the diet. "We had no heat or electricity and had to leave for 5 days," she says. "I went to my mother's house, bringing what I could from my freezer, and I ate the stuff I had. It was tough—I had a lot more on my mind than following the diet to a T".

After surviving Sandy and its very real distractions, Mary says she knew she had found a diet she could follow "anytime, anyplace, and for a long, long time."

The key to the 2 Day, Mary's way:

- ▶ **She savored big cups of vegetable soup.** "The soup really saved me," says Mary. "I ate it for lunch most every day, tossing in tons of vegetables, which I didn't really eat before going on the diet: celery, carrots, onions, string beans, corn, squash—whatever I had. And it filled me up and made me feel virtuous and veggie-loving. It really kept me on the diet despite all my distractions."
- ▶ **She cut back on meat—and embraced spinach.** "I love the meat loaf and spinach recipe," says Mary. "It is delicious—and I don't even like spinach! I'm becoming a veggie lover, which is astonishing to me—and so good for my diet."

CHAPTER 7

Level 2: The Mix and Match Plan

More than 150 quick and easy meals, including restaurant and frozen meal options, give you the freedom to choose your favorites every day of the week.

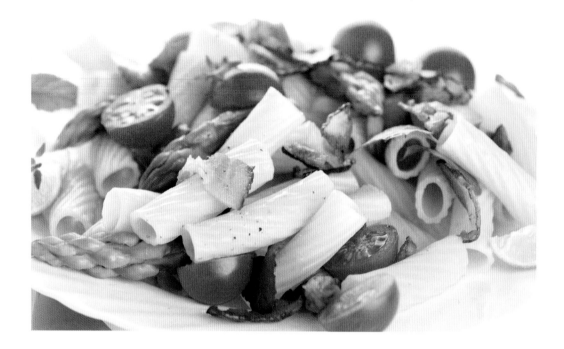

Whether you've already spent some time on Level 1 or whether Level 2 is your first foray into the 2 Day Diabetes Diet, you're going to love the flexibility of this plan. Get ready for options, options, and more options. Rather than follow a set menu of choices, Level 2 allows you to mix and match your meal choices as you see fit. You'll find all of the choices from Level 1, plus much, much more.

Registered dietitian Erin Palinski-Wade has adapted this eating plan to please your modern tastes, to fit your busy modern schedule, and to appeal to your oh-so-finicky modern family. Vegetarian? We've got you covered. Short on time? Not to worry—opt for something from a grab-and-go list. And as our test panelists discovered, you won't have to make two separate meals—one for you, one for your spouse or significant other plus your family. You'll be sitting around the table together, tucking into hearty meals like Round Steak Chili (page 180) and enjoying refreshing dishes like Summer Garden Soup (page 186) and zesty Cherry-Tumeric Yogurt (page 249). Everyone in your family will love the food—and you'll love the ease of preparation and feel great knowing that your loved ones are reaping the same health benefits as you, without giving it a second thought.

Everyone in your family will love the food.

What to Do on Level 2

If you're following the Mix and Match Plan, all you need to do is choose the right foods from the right lists on the right days.

▸ **On your Power Burn Days:** Choose three meals and one snack from the Power Burn list of meal options on pages 124 to 130. On any given day you can choose any combination of breakfast, lunch, dinner, and snack from the Power Burn lists; you can have a different combo every day or just stick to your favorites. Just be sure that on each Power Burn Day, you eat one breakfast, one lunch, one dinner, and one snack choice from the Power Burn list.

▸ **On your Nourishment Days:** Choose three meals and one snack from the Nourishment list of meal options on pages 131 to 138. Two days a week on Nourishment Days, choose from the list of treats on page 138. You can even eat, say, a lunch option for breakfast and the breakfast meal for lunch.

That's it. Pretty simple, right?

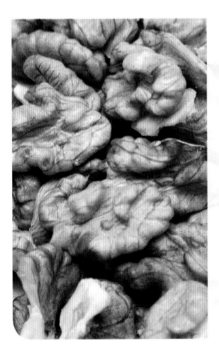

SUPERFOOD SPOTLIGHT: Walnuts

The most widespread tree nut in the world, walnuts contain the polyunsaturated fatty acid called alpha-linolenic acid, which has been shown to lower inflammation.[1] The L-arginine, omega-3s, fiber, vitamin E, and other phytochemicals found in walnuts and other tree nuts make them crazy potent: Scientists have found them to have antioxidant, anticancer, antiviral, and anti-high-cholesterol actions. These powers can help stop and reverse the progression of chronic conditions such as diabetes and heart disease.[2] Walnuts can go rancid once they're removed from their shells, so pile up a bowl of pretty whole walnuts in the center of your kitchen table and put a nutcracker next to it—when you're hungry, stop there first. Just taking the time to crack the nuts can help you slow down and savor your snack, so your belly has more time to register the food and you feel full with fewer calories.

Ensure Your Success

Now that you are in the driver's seat, so to speak, you'll want to plan ahead. Especially on your Power Burn days, you want to make sure you have all the ingredients on hand to make your meals count; because these days are so low-calorie, it's important to get as much nutrition as possible in every bite. (Pictured here is one full day's worth of Power Burn meals; you can see that you won't starve on these days, if you plan them right!). So before you get started on Level 2, we recommend you:

▶ **Decide which days will be your Power Burn Days.**
Remember: Follow the Power Burn meal plan 2 days per week and the Nourishment meal plan 5 days each week. You can choose any 2 days to be your Power Burn Days; they can be spaced out during the week or scheduled back-to-back.

▶ **Eat three meals and one snack each day,** choosing from the meal options listed.

▶ **Plan on having two treats a week,** on any Nourishment Days you choose. Choose them from the provided treats list and enjoy them in addition to your snack for those days.

▶ **Read through the recipes and meal options carefully.**
Make a list of which foods you'd like to try, and write out at least 1 week's meal plan. Check the kitchen cabinets, make a shopping list, look at your schedule, and decide when you can do the cooking. You don't have to prepare the whole week's menu in advance (though you could, if you're the ambitious type). But you do want to be sure that you have all the ingredients on hand, and time in your schedule to put each meal together. In some cases, of course, you can just assemble a wrap or cook an omelet when you need it. Other options require more prep work and cooking time, so factor that into your planning.

Ready? Let's get cooking.

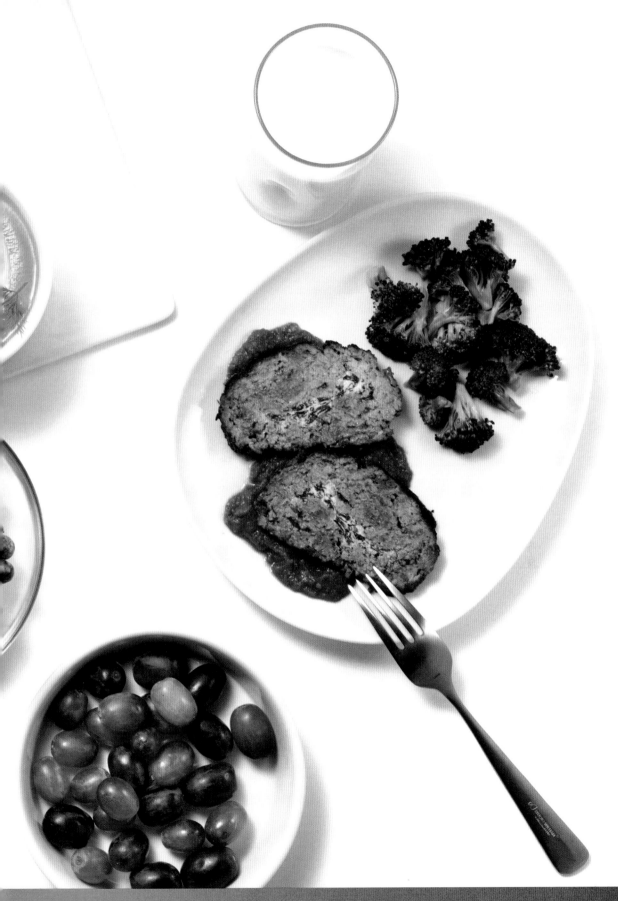

*Power Burn Food Options

On Power Burn Days, choose from these lists for your breakfast, lunch, dinner, and snack. Eat only these choices, and drink water or unsweetened beverages. Unless otherwise noted, you should eat 1 serving of a recipe per meal. (Recipes are provided in Chapter 9.) Note that meals and recipes should use 2% milk and low-fat yogurt. In general, this should be plain yogurt but flavored yogurts are okay if artificially sweetened. Added sugar in yogurt is a no-no.

Breakfast Choices (choose one per day):

EGG DISHES

Omelet made with 2 egg whites and ½ cup cooked onions and peppers, cooked in cooking spray. Serve with 1 cup 2% plain yogurt (130 calories per cup).

Mushroom Quiche (page 173). Serve topped with ½ cup diced tomatoes, and 1 cup 2% milk

1 hard-boiled egg, 1 tomato sliced and topped with pepper and salt, 1 cup 2% milk

MEAT DISHES

1 ounce Canadian bacon, with ½ cup frozen spinach, cooked, 1 cup 2% milk

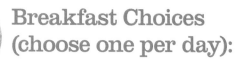

1 ounce low-fat turkey sausage (3 grams of fat or less), 1 egg over easy, 1 cup 2% milk

1 ounce low-fat turkey sausage (3 grams of fat or less), 1 Laughing Cow Light Cheese wedge, 1 cup 2% milk

FISH DISHES

1 ounce smoked salmon (can substitute poached or grilled), ½ cup roasted asparagus, 1 cup 2% milk

VEGETARIAN DISHES

Baked Tomato (page 240), with 1 cup 2% milk

1 cup low-fat yogurt sprinkled with cinnamon, ½ cup steamed broccoli topped with 1 ounce low-fat cheese, melted

1 cup **Yogurt Vegetable Dip (page 248),** 1 cup baby carrots, 1 low-fat string cheese

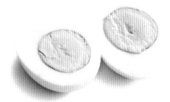

GRAB-AND-GO DISHES

1 pre-cooked hard-boiled egg, 1 cup raw carrot sticks, 1 cup 2% milk

1 low-fat string cheese, 1 medium tomato, sliced, 1 cup 2% plain yogurt

Lunch Choices (choose one per day):

SALADS

Warm Green Vegetable Salad with Garlic and Ginger (page 191). Serve with 8 ounces prepared bouillon (from recipe or cube) and 1 cup 2% plain yogurt topped with 1 cup fresh strawberries.

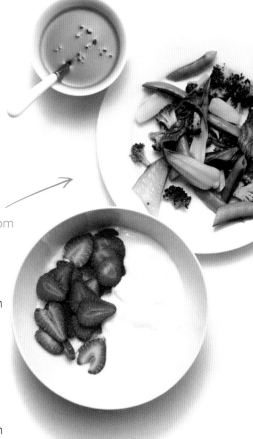

1 cup fresh mixed greens with 1 tablespoon vinegar and 1 teaspoon olive oil, 1 medium apple, and 1 cup bouillon (any flavor)

1 cup garden salad topped with 15 raisins, 1 tablespoon silvered almonds, and 2 tablespoons low-fat dressing with 1 cup bouillon (any flavor)

1 cup fresh mixed greens with 1 tablespoon vinegar and 1 teaspoon olive oil, 1 medium apple, and 1 cup bouillon (any flavor)

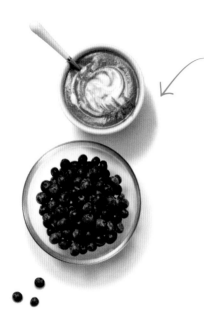

SOUPS

Carrot Soup with Dill (page 185), served with 1 cup fresh blueberries

1 serving (8 ounces) **Bouillon Vegetable Soup (page 183),** plus ½ banana topped with 2 teaspoons peanut butter

Bouillon Vegetable Soup (page 183), 1 cup watermelon, 1 tablespoon sunflower seeds

Bouillon Fruit Stew (page 250), garden salad topped with 2 tablespoons light dressing

Baked Apple (page 179), with **Bouillon Vegetable Soup (page 000)**

VEGETARIAN DISHES

2 large celery stalks topped with 2 teaspoons natural nut butter, with 1 cup fresh berries and 8 ounces bouillon

Roasted Asparagus and Red Pepper with Parmesan (page 234), served with 8 ounces bouillon and 1 medium apple

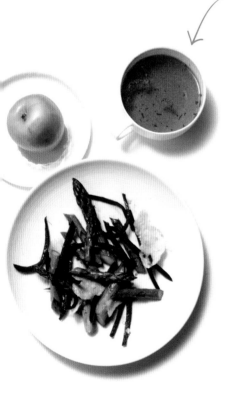

1 cup bouillon (any flavor), 1 cup raw carrots dipped in 2 tablespoons hummus, 1 medium plum

Sautéed kale in 1 teaspoon olive oil, 8 ounces bouillon, 1 serving of berries

1 serving **Steamed Sesame Spinach (page 233),** served with 8 ounces prepared bouillon and 1 cup 2% plain yogurt topped with 1 cup fresh blackberries

1 serving **Roasted Carrots with Rosemary (page 237)** with 8 ounces bouillon and Yogurt Fruit Dip (page 248) with 1 medium apple, sliced

Mashed Cauliflower (page 240), 8 ounces bouillon, 15 grapes

1 cup bouillon (any flavor), 1 cup grilled eggplant, ½ cup pineapple, 6 almonds

GRAB AND GO

1 can Progresso French Onion soup served with 1 medium apple topped with 2 teaspoons natural almond butter

Dinner Choices
(choose one per day):

MEAT DISHES

½ serving **Spinach-Stuffed Meat Loaf (page 199),** served with ½ cup steamed broccoli and 1 cup 2% milk

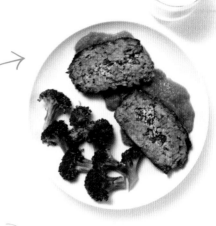

Grilled Chicken Kabobs (page 204), ½ cup zucchini cooked with cooking spray over ¼ cup whole-grain pasta, 1 cup 2% milk

1 cup steamed spinach, 2 ounces grilled chicken breast with 1 cup 2% yogurt, and 1 ½ cups of **Chili Popcorn (page 247)**

2 servings **Roasted Carrots with Rosemary (page 237),** with 2 ounces broiled flank steak served on 1 slice of reduced-calorie bread, and 1 cup 2% milk

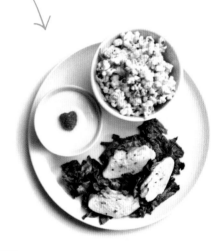

2 servings **Warm Green Vegetable Salad (page 191),** served with 2 ounces grilled chicken, tossed with ¼ cup cooked whole-wheat pasta, and 1 cup 2% milk

Chicken breast (3 ounces raw, to equal 2 ounces cooked) sautéed in cooking spray with 1 tablespoon soy sauce and 2 cups mixed vegetables (mushrooms, onions, peppers, water chestnuts), served over ¼ cup wild rice, with 1 cup 2% milk

2 ounces pork tenderloin (broiled or grilled), ½ cup pumpkin (cut in chunks and boiled), 1 cup fresh greens with lemon juice and salt/pepper to taste, 1 cup 2% milk

2 ounces sirloin steak with 1 cup roasted and mashed turnips, 1 cup 2% yogurt topped with ¼ cup whole-grain cereal

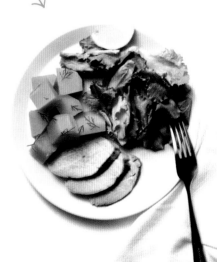

Turkey burger salad: 2 ounces grilled turkey breast burger over 2 cups spinach leaves, with ½ serving of **Baked Sweet Potato "Fries" (page 238)** (but use cooking spray instead of oil), 1 cup 2% milk

2 ounces grilled or broiled chicken or flank steak, 1 cup steamed broccoli, 1 cup 2% milk

Open-face turkey sandwich: 2 ounces turkey breast on top of 1 slice light bread, with 1 cup **Mashed Cauliflower (page 240)** and 1 cup 2% milk

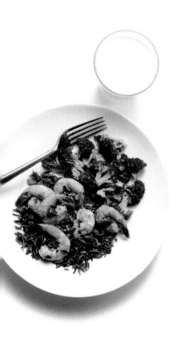

FISH DISHES

½ serving **Baked Cod Casserole with Potatoes, Tomatoes, and Arugula (page 214),** served with 1 ½ cups fresh greens topped with 2 tablespoons shredded low-fat cheese and 2 tablespoons red wine vinegar, 1 cup 2% milk

⅓ cup **Zippy Shrimp (page 218),** served with ¼ cup prepared wild rice and 1 cup steamed broccoli, 1 cup 2% milk

2 ounces broiled salmon, 1 cup steamed green beans, 1 cup 2% milk

½ serving **Sunshine Halibut (page 212),** served with ½ cup mushrooms and ½ cup red bell peppers sautéed in cooking spray, mixed with ¼ cup prepared wild rice, 1 cup 2% milk

1 cup yogurt topped with ¼ cup whole-grain cereal, 2 ounces tuna steak with ½ cup mushrooms and ½ cup collard greens sautéed in cooking spray

2 servings **Steamed Sesame Spinach (page 233),** served with 2 ounces salmon, ¼ cup prepared bulgur, and 1 cup 2% milk

VEGETARIAN DISHES

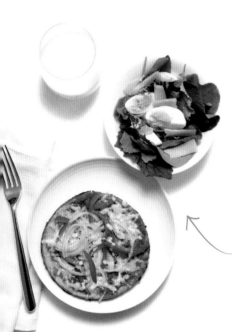

Portabella Mushroom Pizza (page 221) with ¼ cup whole-grain pasta and 1 cup 2% milk

1 cup **Yogurt Vegetable Dip (page 248)** with 1 cup raw carrots, ½ cup steamed edamame, **Baked Tomato (page 240)**

Pita Pizza (page 223), 1 ½ cups fresh salad greens topped with 1 hard-boiled egg and 2 tablespoons shredded low-fat cheese and 2 tablespoons red wine vinegar, 1 cup 2% milk

GRAB AND GO

½ cup canned tuna in water, drained, over 2 cups pre-made, bagged mixed salad greens, served with 3 whole-grain crackers and 1 cup 2% milk

✳ Power Burn Snack Choices
(choose one per day):

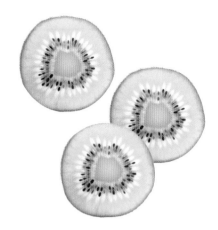

1 cup grapes, purple or green

1 medium orange

2 small plums

¾ cup pineapple

4 apricots

1 cup berries

10 cherries

3 dates

½ grapefruit

½ cup mango

½ cup melon

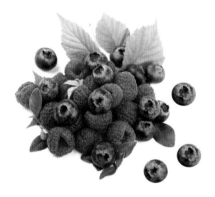

1 medium peach or nectarine

1 medium pear

½ cup unsweetened applesauce

8 dried apricot halves (no sugar added)

2 tablespoons dried cherries, dried cranberries,
   or raisins (no sugar added)

3 prunes

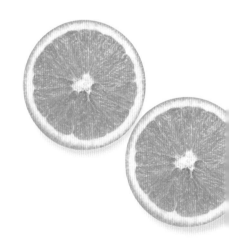

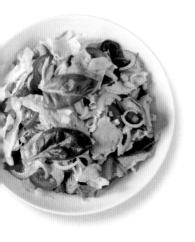

✳ Power Burn Restaurant Options

Especially on your 2 Power Burn Days, it's best to eat at home whenever possible to help you stay on track with your meal plan. (Remember, you can always swap a Power Burn Day with a Nourishment Day as long as each week includes 2 of the former and 5 of the latter.) However, if you can't avoid a restaurant visit, the following options will help you stay on track.

Salad with 3 ounces grilled/boiled/steamed lean protein (the size of a deck of cards) with vinegar and oil on the side (add no more than 1 teaspoon of olive oil; no croutons/cheese/blue cheese crumbles, nuts, etc.)

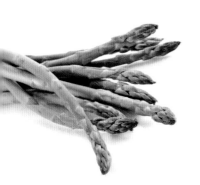

Garden salad with vinegar and 1 teaspoon olive oil with a cup of bouillon on the side or a side of fresh fruit

Steamed vegetables with a side of fresh fruit and/or a cup of bouillon

½ cup low-fat or fat-free cottage cheese with fruit

Grilled, steamed, boiled, or broiled lean protein such as fish or chicken (3 ounces) with a side of steamed vegetables

Omelet with 2 or 3 eggs (or egg whites) and vegetables with a side of fresh fruit

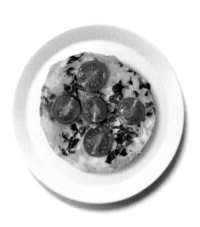

Smoothie made with 2% milk, fruit, and ice (but no additional added sugars or ingredients)

Steamed edamame with sea salt

Broth-based vegetable soup (vegetables must be nonstarchy and soup should not contain any noodles or rice). If soup contains lean protein, remember to count this toward your protein servings for the day.

1 cup 2% plain yogurt with 1 serving fresh fruit

✱ Nourishment Day Food Options

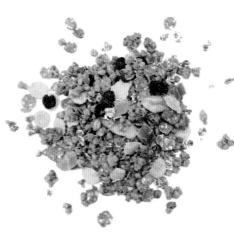

Breakfast Choices (choose one per day):

YOGURT OPTIONS

Yogurt parfait made with 1 cup low-fat plain yogurt, ½ cup whole-grain cereal, and 1 cup blackberries, topped with 1 tablespoon chopped walnuts

1 cup 2% yogurt layered with ⅛ cup granola, 1 tablespoon chopped almonds, 1 cup berries

SMOOTHIES

Blueberry Smoothie (page 252) and 1 slice whole-grain toast with 2 teaspoons nut butter

BREADS, CEREALS, PANCAKES, AND WAFFLES

Peanut Butter Tortilla (page 174), 1 cup low-fat plain yogurt

½ cup whole-grain cereal with ½ cup 2% milk, ½ cup low-fat plain yogurt layered with 3 dates and 1 tablespoon chopped peanuts

½ whole-grain English muffin topped with 2 teaspoons nut butter, ½ cup pineapple, and 1 cup 2% milk

½ cup steel-cut oats topped with 1 tablespoon chopped pecans, cinnamon, and sliced apple, 1 cup 2% milk

½ cup whole-grain cereal with ½ cup 2% milk, ½ cup low-fat yogurt layered with 3 dates and 1 tablespoon chopped peanuts

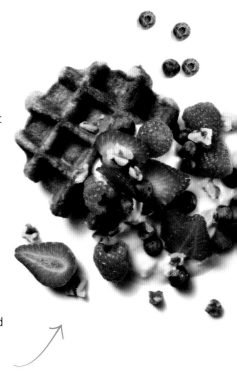

1 whole-grain waffle topped with 1 cup berries, 1 cup low-fat plain yogurt topped with 1 tablespoon chopped walnuts

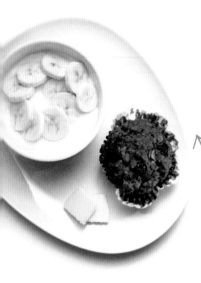

1 ½ cups puffed wheat cereal with 1 cup 2% milk, topped with 1 tablespoon slivered almonds, 1 serving berries

1 whole-grain pancake topped with 1 teaspoon trans-fat-free margarine, 1 peach, 1 cup 2% milk

1 Blueberry Muffin (page 176) with 1 teaspoon trans-fat-free butter spread, 1 cup 2% yogurt topped with ½ banana, sliced

1 VitaMuffin with 1 teaspoon trans-fat-free spread, 1 cup 2% milk, ½ banana

VEGETARIAN DISHES

Banana Toast (page 174), 1 cup low-fat plain yogurt

Baked Apple (page 179), 1 cup low-fat plain yogurt topped with ¼ cup granola

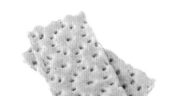

2 Wasa crackers with 2 teaspoons nut butter, ½ cup unsweetened applesauce, 1 cup milk

6 whole-grain crackers with 2 tablespoons hummus, 1 cup yogurt with 1 cup melon

Lunch and Dinner Options (choose one per day):

SANDWICHES

Wrap made with one 12" whole-grain tortilla, 5 ounces deli turkey breast, ½ cup sliced raw hot peppers, ¼ cup sliced onion, ¼ cup diced tomato, and 2 tablespoons hummus, served with 1 cup garden salad and 1 tablespoon dressing on the side

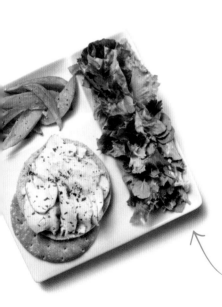

5 ounces turkey breast grilled and served on 1 Arnold's Sandwich Thin and 1 serving **Baked Sweet Potato "Fries" (page 238)** or 1 serving frozen baked sweet potato fries (such as Ian's or Alexa brand), with 2 cups salad greens and 1 tablespoon vinaigrette dressing

6" pita stuffed with 4 ounces grilled chicken breast, 2 tablespoons hummus, and ½ cup roasted red peppers, served with **Baked Tomato (page 240)**

4 ounces sliced turkey breast, 1 ounce low-fat cheese on
2 slices whole-grain bread with 1 teaspoon mayo (or
1 tablespoon light mayo), 2 cups garden salad with
2 tablespoons light vinaigrette dressing

5 ounces sliced chicken breast on 2 slices whole-grain
bread topped with ½ cup roasted red peppers and
2 tablespoons hummus, 1 cup side salad with
1 tablespoon dressing

SOUPS

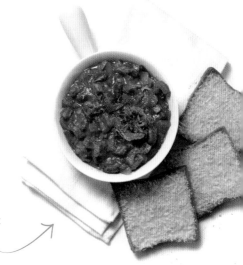

1 serving **Round Steak Chili (page 180),** served with
3 slices reduced-calorie light bread, toasted and topped
with 2 teaspoons trans-fat-free spread, 1 teaspoon garlic
powder, and 4 tablespoons Parmesan cheese (spread
evenly over each slice of bread and toast until melted)

MEAT DISHES

1 serving **Summer Garden Soup (page 186),** served with
5 ounces broiled pork tenderloin, 3 ounces sweet potato
topped with 1 teaspoon trans-fat-free spread, ½ cup
prepared collard greens sautéed in 1 teaspoon olive oil

1 serving **Curried Chicken Dinner (page 205),** with 1 serving
Bulgur with Spring Vegetables (page 242)

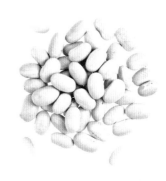

5 ounces flank steak, broiled, topped with 1 cup
mushrooms/onions sautéed in 1 teaspoon olive oil,
3 ounces sweet potato with 1 teaspoon trans-fat-free
spread

5 ounces sautéed chicken breast in 2 teaspoons olive
oil with garlic, 1 cup prepared cannellini beans, 1 cup
steamed broccoli

2 servings **Roasted Asparagus and Red Pepper with
Parmesan (page 234),** served with 5 ounces center-cut
pork chop, ⅔ cup couscous

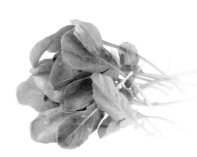

4 ounces grilled turkey burger on whole-grain bun topped
with 1 ounce low-fat/fat-free cheese, served with 2 cups
garden salad with 2 tablespoons dressing

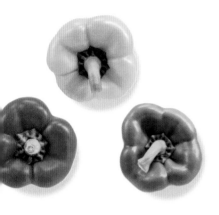

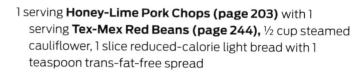

1 serving **Honey-Lime Pork Chops (page 203)** with 1 serving **Tex-Mex Red Beans (page 244)**, ½ cup steamed cauliflower, 1 slice reduced-calorie light bread with 1 teaspoon trans-fat-free spread

1 serving **Carrot Soup with Dill (page 185),** served with 3 ounces grilled chicken breast, ½ cup spinach sautéed in 1 teaspoon olive oil, 1 cup cooked cannellini beans

2 servings **Warm Green Vegetable Salad with Garlic and Ginger (page 191),** served with 5 ounces grilled chicken and 6 ounces sweet potato topped with 2 teaspoons trans-fat-free spread

2 servings **Roasted Carrots with Rosemary (page 237),** served with 5 ounces broiled flank steak, one 6-ounce baked potato, 2 teaspoons trans-fat-free spread

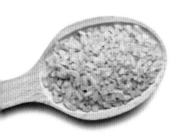

2 servings **Baked Tomato (page 240)** with 3 ounces grilled chicken breast sautéed in 2 teaspoons olive oil, served with ⅔ cup quinoa

5 ounces broiled pork tenderloin, 1 cup mashed sweet potato topped with 1 teaspoon trans-fat-free spread, 1 cup Brussels sprouts sautéed in 1 teaspoon olive oil

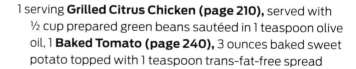

1 serving **Caribbean Chicken (page 206),** served with ¾ cup prepared wild rice, 1 ½ cups fresh greens topped with ¼ cup shredded low-fat cheese, 2 tablespoons light ranch dressing

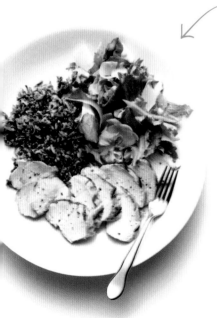

1 serving **Grilled Citrus Chicken (page 210),** served with ½ cup prepared green beans sautéed in 1 teaspoon olive oil, 1 **Baked Tomato (page 240)**, 3 ounces baked sweet potato topped with 1 teaspoon trans-fat-free spread

1 serving **Flank Steak with Red Onions (page 200),** served with ¾ cup steamed kale topped with 2 tablespoons reduced-fat Parmesan cheese and 1 serving **Baked Sweet Potato "Fries" (page 238)**

1 serving **Bulgur with Spring Vegetables (page 242)** with 1 serving **Curried Chicken Dinner (page 205)**

Healthy Chicken Parmesan (page 209) over a bed of 1 cup prepared spinach, steamed

FISH DISHES

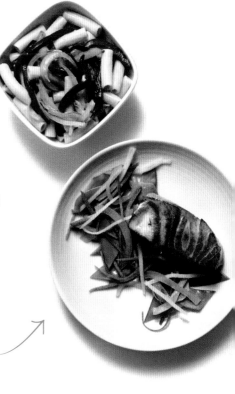

2 servings **Tabbouleh (page 243),** served with
5 ounces broiled flounder

1 serving **Baked Cod Casserole with Potatoes,
Tomatoes, and Arugula (page 214),** served with
1 serving **Tex-Mex Red Beans (page 244)**

¾ cup **Zippy Shrimp (page 218),** served over 2 cups fresh
spinach leaves topped with 2 tablespoons vinaigrette and
1 cup prepared wild rice

2 servings **Creamy Greens Soup (page 188),** served with
5 ounces grilled tuna steak, ½ cup steamed broccoli,
⅓ cup cooked quinoa

1 serving **Asian Steamed Fish Fillets with Vegetable Sticks
(page 217),** served with 1 cup prepared brown rice noodles
tossed with 1 teaspoon olive oil and ½ cup prepared red
peppers and onions sautéed in 1 teaspoon olive oil

5 ounces salmon filet, grilled and served with ⅔ cup whole-
grain couscous and 1 cup collard greens sautéed in
2 teaspoons olive oil

2 servings **Tex-Mex Red Beans (page 244),** served with
3 ounces broiled tilapia

Stir-fry made with 5 ounces shrimp, 1 cup peppers/
onions/mushrooms cooked in 2 teaspoons olive oil, and
1 tablespoon soy sauce, served over ⅔ cup brown rice

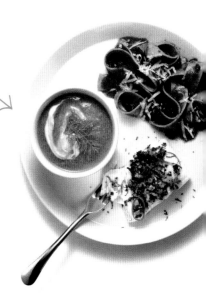

1 serving of **Sunshine Halibut (page 212),** served with
1 serving **Carrot Soup with Dill (page 185)** and 1 cup
whole-wheat pasta topped with ¼ cup tomato sauce,
2 tablespoons reduced-fat Parmesan cheese, and
1 teaspoon olive oil

1 serving **Salmon on a Bed of Greens (page 211),** served
with 1 serving **Summer Garden Soup (page 186)**

2 servings **Steamed Sesame Spinach (page 233),** served
with 5 ounces grilled salmon and 2 slices whole-grain
toast topped with 2 teaspoons trans-fat-free spread

Walnut-Encrusted Tilapia (page 215), served with 1 cup
steamed wax beans and ½ cup prepared wild rice

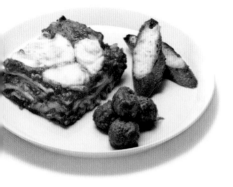

Vegetarian Options

2 servings **Pita Pizza (page 223),** 1 cup fresh garden salad topped with 4 ounces grilled chicken breast, sliced, and 2 tablespoons vinaigrette, 1 small breadstick

12" whole-grain tortilla topped with 5 ounces low-fat mozzarella cheese, ½ cup tomato sauce, ½ cup mushrooms and onions cooked in 2 teaspoons olive oil

1 serving **New Mexican Green Chili (page 182),** served with ½ cup steamed carrots topped with 1 teaspoon trans-fat-free spread, 1 small whole-grain dinner roll

1 serving **Bean and Vegetable Tostadas (page 220),** served with 1 ½ cups fresh greens topped with 1 cup extra-firm light tofu lightly pan-fried in 1 teaspoon olive oil and 2 tablespoons light vinaigrette; ½ cup steamed edamame

1 serving **Eggplant Lasagna (page 224)** served with four 1" vegetarian meatballs and two slices of a baguette, topped with butter spray and 1 tablespoon Parmesan cheese and toasted

1 serving **Barley Risotto with Asparagus and Mushrooms (page 228),** served with ¾ cup low-fat cottage cheese and 2 Wasa crackers

2 servings **Southwestern Black Bean Salad (page 192)** with 1 vegetable burger served over 2 cups fresh spinach leaves with 2 tablespoons light vinaigrette dressing

1 serving **Couscous-Stuffed Peppers (page 227),** served with 1 cup extra-firm light tofu tossed with ¼ cup sweet onion and ¼ cup red bell pepper stir-fried in 1 teaspoon olive oil and low-sodium soy sauce

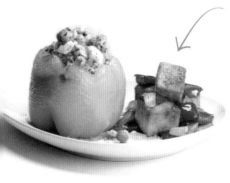

1 serving **Cold Sesame Noodles and Vegetables (page 232)** mixed with 2 cups extra-firm light tofu lightly fried in 1 teaspoon olive oil and served with a side of steamed Brussels sprouts

GRAB AND GO

6 large pre-cooked shrimp, chilled, served over 2 cups fresh spinach leaves topped with 2 tablespoons vinaigrette and 1 cup prepared wild rice

✳ Nourishment Snack Options
(choose one per day):

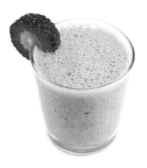

SMOOTHIES
Black Cherry Smoothie (page 251)

Apple-Cinnamon Smoothie (page 250)

Blueberry Smoothie (page 252)

Mango Smoothie (page 252)

FRUIT

Sliced apple topped with cinnamon, 1 cup 2% milk

1 cup purple or green grapes

1 medium orange

¾ cup pineapple

2 plums, 1 cup 2% milk

1 kiwifruit, 1 cup 2% milk

1 nectarine, 1 cup 2% milk

½ banana , 1 cup 2% milk

15 red grapes, 1 cup 2% milk

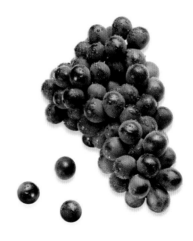

YOGURT

1 cup low-fat yogurt topped with 3 dates and 1 teaspoon
  ground cinnamon

Cherry-Turmeric Yogurt (page 249)

1 cup watermelon, 1 cup low-fat yogurt

1 orange, 1 cup low-fat yogurt

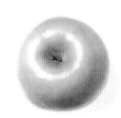

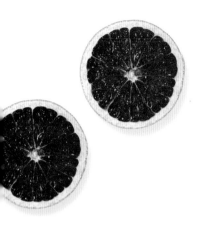

Parfait made with alternating layers of low-fat yogurt and sliced honeydew melon

1 cup low-fat yogurt topped with 1 teaspoon cocoa powder, 1 pear

Yogurt Fruit Dip (page 248), peach cut into slices for dipping

1 cup low-fat yogurt topped with 4 apricots and sprinkled with cinnamon

1 cup low-fat yogurt topped with 2 tablespoons raisins

1 cup 2% yogurt with 1 cup strawberries

Yogurt parfait made by layering 1 cup low-fat yogurt with ½ banana, sliced, and topped with cinnamon

½ grapefruit, 1 cup low-fat yogurt

2 tangerines, 1 cup low-fat yogurt

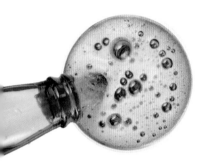

* Nourishment Treat Options (choose two per week):

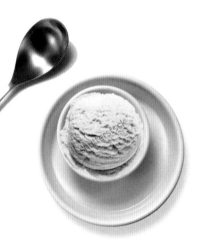

1-ounce bag baked chips

1 ounce dark chocolate (60% cacao or above)

12 ounces light beer

4 ounces red or white wine

1 ½ ounces liquor (mixed with sugar-free mixer)

½ cup ice cream

½ scone (small)

1 small (2"-diameter) cookie

❋ Frozen Meal Options

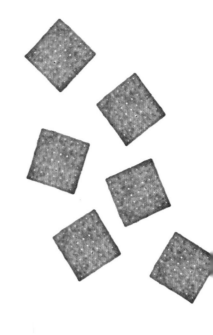

In general, it's best to cook your own food. That's because there's no frozen meal that is perfectly calibrated with the 2 Day Diabetes Diet. Many, for instance, are very high in sodium. Some are also low in vegetables and other wholesome nutrients. That said, these tend to be more balanced than most fast food options. . .and are certainly better than not eating at all. (Remember, you want to keep your blood sugar balanced and not let yourself get hungry!) That's why Erin went through the grocery store and read the labels, finding the healthiest frozen meals and pairing them with grab-and-go foods (where she recommends steamed vegetables, you can often buy them frozen and steam them in the microwave alongside your frozen entrée). These are best used on Nourishment days.

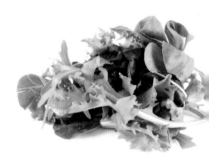

Organic Bistro's Wild Salmon (with cranberry pilaf and walnut broccoli), paired with 2 cups bagged salad greens topped with 1 hard-boiled egg, 2 tablespoons Parmesan cheese, and 1 tablespoon light vinaigrette dressing

Organic Bistro's Southwest Style Grass-Fed Beef, served with 1 cup steamed edamame and ½ cup steamed carrots

Organic Bistro's Wild Alaska Salmon, served with ½ cup steamed broccoli topped with 1 slice (1 ounce) low-fat Cheddar cheese, melted

Kashi Frozen Entrées Lemongrass Coconut Chicken, paired with 2 cups bagged salad greens topped with 1 hard-boiled egg, 2 tablespoons Parmesan cheese, and 2 tablespoons light vinaigrette

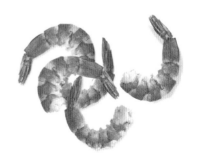

Kashi Frozen Entrées Lime Cilantro Shrimp, served with 1 cup salad greens topped with ½ cup canned crab meat, drained and mixed with 1 tablespoon light mayonnaise

Lean Cuisine Salmon with Basil, served with 6 whole-grain crackers topped with 2 teaspoons peanut butter and ¼ cup soy nuts

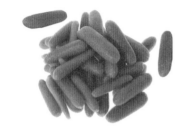

Lean Cuisine Glazed Chicken, served with 1 cup Brussels sprouts sautéed in 1 teaspoon olive oil and 2 Laughing Cow Light Cheese wedges

Lean Cuisine Roasted Turkey Breast with green beans, served with ½ cup soy nuts and 1 cup raw carrots

Healthy Choice Café Steamers Grilled Chicken & Roasted Red Pepper Alfredo Sauce, served with 1 cup Amy's Vegetable Barley soup and 1 ounce low-fat string cheese

Healthy Choice Cajun Style Chicken & Shrimp, served with 1 cup steamed cauliflower and ½ cup soy nuts

2 Amy's Black Bean/Vegetable Enchiladas, served with 3 ounces grilled chicken breast on top of 1 cup steamed spinach leaves

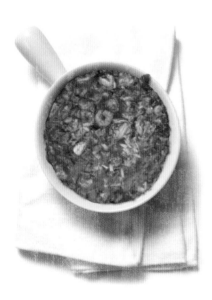

Amy's Brown Rice, Black-eyed Peas & Veggies Bowl, served with 1 cup low-fat cottage cheese and 1 cup sliced cucumber

Amy's Garden Vegetable Lasagna, served with 3 ounces turkey meatballs (store bought or homemade) and ¾ cup steamed string beans

Trader Joe's Trader Ming's BBQ Chicken Teriyaki (2 cups), served with 1 cup onions/peppers sautéed in 2 teaspoons olive oil

½ container Trader Joe's Chicken Serenada, paired with 2 cups Amy's Organic Low-Fat Vegetable Barley soup

Seeds of Change Spicy Yucatan Frijoles, served with 1 cup salad greens topped with ¼ cup shredded low-fat cheese and 2 tablespoons light vinaigrette dressing, 1 low-fat string cheese

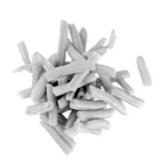

1 cup Amy's Organic Low-Fat Vegetable Barley Soup, served with 1 ½ cups salad greens topped with 2 ounces grilled chicken and 2 tablespoons balsamic vinegar, 1 cup 2% milk

THE 2 DAY WAY
Joyce Slavin

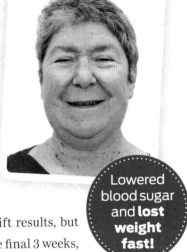

Lowered blood sugar and lost weight fast!

Making strides. That's what Joyce Slavin has been doing—literally as well as figuratively. The 58-year-old former special education teacher from New Rochelle, New York, joined our test panel to gain more control over her type 2 diabetes as well as drop some pounds.

And she did exactly that. Within just 3 weeks, her fasting blood sugar was down by 32 points (a 22 percent decrease) and her weight by 7 pounds. She was thrilled with those swift results, but then surprised herself when she dropped 2 more pounds in the final 3 weeks, in part by extending her daily walks and quickening her pace.

"I walk every day, for at least an hour a day, with a friend," says Joyce. "Neither of us is working now, so we typically walk for as long as we want—sometimes up to 2 hours. As I progressed on the diet, though, I found that I was walking faster and longer on the days my friend wasn't able to go with me. I was getting better, feeling lighter, fitter, and more energetic. I really believe the walking saved me."

Saved her? From what? "Chinese food," squeals Joyce—"I could eat it three times a day, 7 days a week!" Joyce doesn't have an oven, just a microwave. But she found the plan easy to follow, despite not having a full kitchen. "I have always watched what I eat, but I tend to yo-yo—lose and then gain again," she says. "Well, not this time. This time, I'm finding it surprisingly easy to stick with the program. The Power Burn Days are especially easy for me, since I don't have to prepare much food—and they work. I've had to add four holes to my belt."

The key to the 2 Day, Joyce's way:

▶ **She exercised for at least an hour a day, every day.** "My walks kept me on track," says Joyce, I felt like I was moving forward every day, and that's because I literally was."

▶ **She celebrated every pound lost with her walking buddy.** "This is a diet you can totally do on your own," says Joyce. "You don't have to pay anyone for the privilege of weighing in with them. But it just helps to share the experience."

CHAPTER 8

Level 3: The Free Range Plan

Create your own meals, even incorporating packaged foods as appropriate. Plus, eat out at fast food, Mexican, Italian, and other restaurants.

Levels 1 and 2 of the 2 Day Diabetes Diet give you all the nutrition and dietary structure you need to live a long and happy life. There will be times, however, when you need more options. Maybe you are planning a large gathering. Maybe you have a business lunch or are sensitive to a certain ingredient. Perhaps it's the holidays or you just generally want to adapt some old family favorites to 2 Day Diabetes Diet eating.

Not to fear: Level 3 is here.

On this level of the 2 Day Diabetes Diet, you have free range. You'll learn how to create your own Power Burn and Nourishment meals with the right balance of nutrients for lasting success. Based on the information on number of servings per meal and serving sizes, you'll be able to adapt the plan as needed.

Make It Work for You

Everything from Levels 1 and 2 works in Level 3, so lean on those menus and food lists to ease your transition into Level 3 eating.

When creating Level 3 meals and menus, keep the following guidelines in mind:

> Plan Power Burn Days separately from Nourishment Days. Remember, your Power Burn Days include many fewer calories and carbs than your Nourishment Days, so they use a completely different meal-planning formula.

> Aim for at least 64 ounces of any of the following fluids every day: club soda, seltzer, coffee (preferably decaf), tea (preferably decaf), and water. We discourage artificially sweetened beverages. Hold yourself to no more than two a week.

> Condiments are not counted in your daily number of servings for fat or veggies, so don't overdo them. Whether it's a Nourishment or a Power Burn Day, hold yourself to 2 daily tablespoons or fewer of ketchup, relish, or soy sauce. Horseradish, mustard, and vinegar, however, are unlimited.

> If you'd like to use cooking oil, count it as one of your fat servings (see "The 2 Day Diabetes Formula" below for guidance). You do

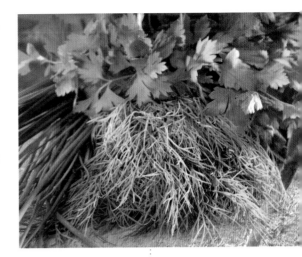

not, however, have to count cooking spray as long as you only lightly spritz the pan.

▸ The following seasonings and spices are unlimited: flavor extracts, garlic, fresh or dried herbs, hot pepper, black or white pepper, pimiento, spices (cayenne pepper, cinnamon, turmeric, cloves, etc.), cooking wine, and lemon or lime juice used in cooking.

▸ As with Levels 1 and 2, consume up to two treats a week—in addition to your snacks, and only on Nourishment Days. Choose from among 1 ounce of baked chips (roughly 15 chips), 1 ounce of dark (60% cacao or higher) chocolate, 12 ounces of light beer, 4 ounces of red or white wine, 1½ ounces of liquor, ½ cup of regular ice cream (free of sugar-loaded mix-ins such as cookie dough), 1 small cookie or scone (2" diameter).

▸ Try to consume a superfood and 1 teaspoon of a super seasoning at least three times a week. (See page 68 for the complete list.)

The 2 Day Diabetes Diet Formula

The following chart will help you build your own Power Burn and Nourishment menus. Just hold true to the number of servings in each food group per day, picking and choosing among the listed options and their serving sizes.

All the ingredients in each type of meal are balanced to ensure you get the optimal fat-burning power and nutritional composition over the course of a day. Remember: The number of servings on Power Burn Days differs from the number on Nourishment Days.

VEGETABLES (4 SERVINGS PER DAY)	FRUIT (2 SERVINGS PER DAY)	MILK (2 SERVINGS PER DAY)	STARCH (½ SERVING ON POWER BURN DAYS; 5 ON NOURISHMENT DAYS
½ c any cooked non-starchy vegetable	1 small apple, kiwifruit, nectarine, orange	1 c 2% milk	1 slice 100% whole-grain bread (or 2 slices reduced- calorie bread)
1 c any raw non-starchy vegetable	4 apricots	1 c soy, coconut, or almond milk	¼ 100% whole-grain bagel
6 oz (¾ c) 100% vegetable juice	½ banana	milk (10 g sugar or less per serving)	½ 100% whole-grain English muffin
	1 c berries	1 c 2% yogurt (plain or artificially sweetened)	One 6" 100% whole-grain tortilla
	10 cherries		One 4" 100% whole-grain pancake
	3 small dates		½ burger or dog 100% whole-grain bun or 6" 100% whole-grain pita
	½ grapefruit		½ c 100% whole-grain pasta, wild rice, cereal, oatmeal, tabbouleh, bulgur, cooked kasha
	15 small grapes (1 c total)		⅓ c brown rice, quinoa, couscous, barley
	1 medium peach, pear		3 Tbsp wheat germ
	½ c cubed melon or mango		1 ½ c puffed cereal
	¾ c pineapple		½ c starchy vegetables (corn, parnsips, peas, mashed potato, yams)
	2 small plums or tangerines		1 c pumpkin or winter squash
	½ c canned fruit, canned in juice		3 oz or ½ medium baked regular or sweet potato
	2 Tbsp dried cherries, cranberries, raisins		⅓ c plantain
	3 prunes		½ cup beans, legumes, or lentils (counts as 1 oz protein and 1 starch serving)
	8 dried apricots		½ cup edamame (counts as 1 oz protein and ½ starch serving)
	1 ½ figs		
	½ c 100% juice (4 oz)		
	⅓ c prune juice (2 ½ oz)		

LEAN PROTEIN (3 OZ ON POWER BURN DAYS; 10 OZ ON NOURISHMENT DAYS)	FAT (1 SERVING ON POWER BURN DAYS; 5 ON NOURISHMENT DAYS	BOUILLON (8 OZ ON POWER BURN DAYS)
1 oz any fish or shellfish	1 tsp cooking oil, margarine, trans-fat-free mayonnaise, butter	Vegetable, chicken, or beef
1 oz lean poultry: skinless poultry breast, Cornish hen, or ground poultry breast	1 Tbsp reduced- fat mayo	
1 oz pork: Canadian bacon, ham, tenderloin, center-cut chop, loin	2 Tbsp mashed avocado or ¼ small avocado	
1 oz beef: flank steak, ground round, roast, round, sirloin, tenderloin (trimmed of fat)	8 black olives or 10 green olives	
1 oz lamb: roast, chop, or leg	1 ½ tsp nut butter	
1 oz low-fat cheese (3 g fat or less per oz)	2 Tbsp hummus	
1 egg	Nuts: 6 almonds or cashews, 3 macadamia nuts, 10 peanuts, 4 pecan halves, 16 pistachios	
2 egg whites or ¼ c egg whites or substitute	1 Tbsp pumpkin, sesame, or sunflower seeds	
1 oz lean lunch meat (roughly 1 slice)	1 Tbsp regular or 2 Tbsp reduced-fat salad dressing	
½ c beans, legumes, or lentils (counts as 1 oz protein and 1 starch serving)		
½ c edamame (counts as 1 oz protein and ½ starch serving)		

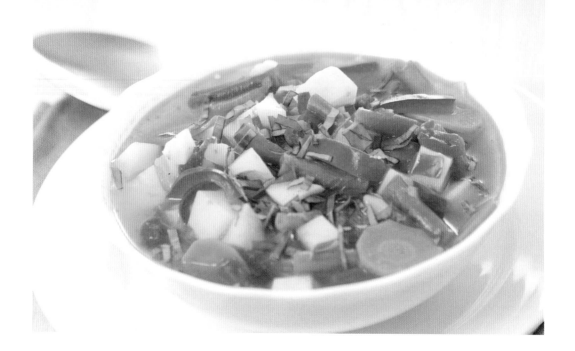

How to Use the Formula to Build Your Meals

It's up to you how you split up your daily vegetable, fruit, fat, protein, and other servings. Just try to spread them out evenly throughout the day. For instance, try not to consume all of your grains at breakfast or all of your protein for dinner. To gain an idea of how to do this, here's a suggestion for how you can break it down meal-by-meal.

Sample Day of Power Burn Eating

BREAKFAST: 1 serving of milk, 1 ounce of protein, 1 vegetable serving

Examples:

6 ounces vegetable juice + 1 cup yogurt + 1 hard-boiled egg

2 scrambled egg whites with ½ cup chopped veggies (bell pepper, onion, tomato) + 1 cup milk

1 ounce smoked salmon + 1 cup sliced cucumbers + 1 cup yogurt

LUNCH: 8 ounces of bouillon, 1 vegetable serving, 1 fruit serving, 1 fat serving

Examples:

Veggie soup made with 8 ounces bouillon and ½ cup cooked veggies
+ 1 ½ teaspoons peanut butter on 1 small apple

Avocado salad made with ¼ small avocado, sliced, 1 cup chopped
tomato and cucumber, ½ cup cubed mango + 8 ounces bouillon

Green smoothie made with ¾ cup frozen pineapple, 8 ounces bouillon,
1 cup raw spinach, 2 tablespoons avocado

DINNER: 2 ounces of protein, ½ serving of whole grains,
2 servings of vegetables, 1 serving of milk

Examples:

2 ounces salmon + ¼ cup wild rice + 1 cup steamed veggies + 1 cup milk

2 ounces grilled, cubed chicken breast mixed with ¼ cup pasta
+ 1 cup steamed veggies + 1 cup milk

2 ounces grilled shrimp served over a bed of steamed greens
+ 1 cup yogurt with ½ slice bread

SNACK: 1 serving of fruit

Sample Day of Nourishment Eating

BREAKFAST: 1 serving of milk, 1 serving of whole grains,
1 serving of fruit, 1 serving of fat

Examples:

1 slice toast with 1 teaspoon margarine + 1 cup berries with 1 cup yogurt

Smoothie made with 1 cup yogurt, 1 cup frozen strawberries, 1 tablespoon
pumpkin seeds and 3 tablespoons wheat germ

Yogurt parfait made with 1 cup yogurt, 1 cup breakfast cereal, ½ sliced
banana, 10 peanuts

LUNCH: 2 servings of vegetables, 2 servings of whole grains, 5 ounces of protein, 2 servings of fat

Examples:

Salad made with 2 cups greens and chopped veggies, 5 ounces smoked salmon, 8 black olives, 1 tablespoon seeds, and 1 cup cooked pasta

1 cup cooked winter squash roasted with ½ cup parsnips and 2 tablespoons cooking oil + turkey and cheese sandwich (3 slices turkey, 1 slice cheese, 2 slices bread)

2 cups chopped tomato, onion, and cucumber salad with 2 teaspoons oil + ½ bagel melt (3 slices turkey, 1 slice cheese melted over 1 slice tomato and bagel)

DINNER: 2 servings of vegetables, 2 servings of whole grains, 5 ounces of protein, 2 servings of fat

Examples:

5 ounces flank steak + ⅔ cup rice + 2 cups salad with 2 teaspoons oil

Stir-fry made with 5 ounces cubed chicken breast, 2 teaspoons oil, 1 cup assorted, chopped stir-fry veggies, and ⅔ cup rice

Bean burrito made with 1 cup beans, 2 ounces cheese, ⅔ cup rice + 2 cups salad with 2 teaspoons oil

SNACK: 1 SERVING OF FRUIT, 1 SERVING OF MILK

Examples:

1 cup yogurt mixed with 1 cup berries

1 cup milk + 1 small apple

1 cup yogurt + ½ grapefruit

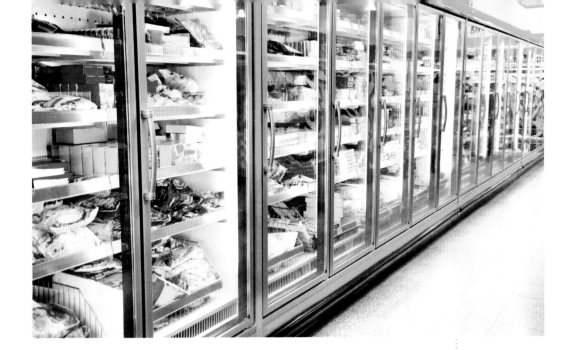

How to Use Packaged Foods

Your Power Burn and Nourishment formulas will help you easily build meals from whole foods. What do you do when you want to work in a packaged meal—one that contains an unknown mix of vegetables, protein, and other foods?

That's where the diabetic exchanges come in. Developed by the American Diabetes and American Dietetic Association, these exchanges group like foods together: vegetables, fruits, starches, fats, proteins, dairy. Sound familiar? It should, because the formula behind the 2 Day Diabetes Diet closely matches up with these exchanges; consider these formulas the 2 Day Diabetes Diet exchanges.

Some packaged foods come with diabetic exchanges listed on the label. If that's the case, just count the servings listed on the package as your starch, vegetable, protein, and so on. If the exchanges are not listed, you'll need to do a little math. You can do this one of two ways.

Method #1: Convert what's listed on the Nutrition Facts label into a serving from one of your food groups. This is a good method if you consume packaged foods only occasionally. To do so, use the following conversions.

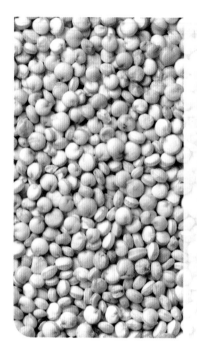

SUPERFOOD SPOTLIGHT: Quinoa

Quinoa tastes like a grain, but it's more closely related to spinach than it is to rice. It also packs a nutrient punch that few other foods, let alone grains, can match. Contrary to most grains, quinoa is a dense source of "complete" protein (14 grams per ½ cup!), boasting all nine essential amino acids. One is lysine, which helps the body absorb all that fabulous fat-burning calcium and also helps produce carnitine, a nutrient responsible for converting fatty acids into energy and helping to lower cholesterol. We know how fiber helps to balance blood sugar levels and keep us fuller longer—quinoa is one of the most fiber-rich grain-like foods, with 2.6 grams per ½ cup. Try it as a replacement for rice or couscous, or use it like tabbouleh, as a base for a Mediterranean cucumber and tomato salad. You can even prepare it for breakfast, instead of grits or oatmeal. Just pour on a little milk and honey, sprinkle with cinnamon, and you have a hearty, protein-rich, nutrition-packed start to your day!

To convert carbohydrate grams to starch servings:

1. Calculate your net carbs:

If a food contains 5 grams of fiber or more:

Total carbohydrate – Half the grams of fiber = Net carbs

In the food label example on page 153, that's

**31 grams of carbohydrate – 3 grams of fiber
= 28 net carbohydrate grams**

If a food contains less than 5 grams of fiber, use the total carbohydrate content as your net carbs:

2. Convert net carb grams to grain/starch servings:

One grain/starch serving = 15 grams of carbohydrates

In the food label example above, that means your 28 net carbs = nearly 2 servings of starch

To convert protein grams to protein ounces/servings:

1 ounce of protein = 7 grams of protein

In the sample label, there are 14 grams of protein, or 2 ounces.

To convert fat grams to fat servings:

1 fat serving = 5 grams of fat

The sample food contains 9 grams of fat, or 2 servings

Method #2: Plan your meals using a formula that matches up with what's listed on packaged foods. This is a good strategy if you consume a lot of packaged foods. Use the following formulas for packaged foods.

For meals on Power Burn Days, try to stay within the following daily totals for these nutrients, all listed in the Nutrition Facts panel of any packaged food:

- 75 grams of carbohydrates
- 42 grams of protein
- 21 grams of fat
- 13 grams of fiber
- 600 to 650 calories (45 percent from carbohydrates, 25 percent from protein, 30 percent from fat)

For meals on Nourishment Days, try to stay within the following daily totals for these nutrients, all listed in the Nutrition Facts panel of any packaged food:

- 185 grams of carbohydrates
- 90 grams of protein
- 45 grams of fat
- 25 to 30 grams of fiber
- 1,500 calories (50 percent from carbohydrates, 25 percent from protein, 25 percent from fat)

It's up to you how you split up those grams within your three meals and one daily snack. Again, just try to spread them out evenly throughout the day. For instance, try not to consume all of your protein at the same meal.

Let's say, for instance, that you are planning a Power Burn dinner. Based on what you've already had for breakfast and lunch and remembering that you want to save some room for snack, you decide you want your dinner to include the following:

- ▶ 25 grams of carbohydrates
- ▶ 24 grams of protein
- ▶ 9 grams of fat
- ▶ 5 grams of fiber

Now compare that to the Nutrition Facts panel for a sandwich you think might make a good dinner.

Nutrition Facts

Serving Size 1 sandwich

Amount per serving

Calories 300   Calories from fat 80

	% Daily Value*
Total Fat 9g	**14**%
Saturated Fat 1g	**5**%
Polyunsaturated Fat 4.5g	
Trans Fat 0g	
Cholesterol 75mg	**25**%
Sodium 350mg	**15**%
Total Carbohydrate 31g	**24**%
Dietary Fiber 6g	
Sugars 10g	
Protein 14g	

*Percent Daily Values are based on a 2,000 calorie diet. Your daily values may be higher or lower depending on your calorie needs.

You'll see that one serving of this sandwich contains 31 grams of carbohydrates, a little more than your "budget" allows. With only 14 grams of protein, though, it's a little short of your goal. Also, at 300 calories, this sandwich contains almost half your daily 650-calorie allotment. So you might choose to make this an open-faced sandwich, leave off one slice of bread, and add a little extra lean meat to boost the protein. Or you might just choose to eat the whole sandwich and just make sure that the snack you eat is higher in protein and lighter in carbs.

Recommended Grab-and-Go Options

We wanted to make this diet as easy to follow as possible. That's why we asked Erin to do a lot of label reading and calculations for you. Here, you'll find recommended packaged meals and bars, along with the number of 2 Day Diabetes Diet exchanges that each one contains.

Soups

Healthy Valley Fat Free Chicken Noodle Vegetable: 1 cup = *1 ½ oz protein, 3 starch*

Amy's Black Bean Vegetable: 1 cup = *1 ½ starch, 1 oz protein*

Amy's Vegetable Barley: 1 cup = *½ starch, ½ vegetable*

Campbell's Healthy Request Chunky Beef Barley: 1 cup = *1 starch, 1 oz protein*

Campbell's Healthy Request Chunky Chicken Noodle: 1 cup = *1 starch, 1 oz protein*

Campbell's Healthy Request Chunky New England Clam Chowder: 1 cup = *1 starch, 1 oz protein, ½ fat*

Campbell's Healthy Request Chunky Vegetable: 1 cup = *1 starch, ½ vegetable*

Campbell's Select Italian Wedding: 1 cup = *1 starch, 1 fat, 1 oz protein*

Healthy Choice Bean and Ham: 1 cup = *1 ½ starch, 1 ½ oz protein*

Healthy Choice Chicken & Dumplings: 1 cup = *1 starch, 1 oz protein, ½ fat*

Healthy Choice Zesty Gumbo: 1 cup = *1 starch, 1 oz protein*

Healthy Choice Garden Vegetable: 1 cup = *1 starch, 1 vegetable, 1 fat*

Progresso Healthy Favorites Chicken Gumbo: 1 cup = *1 starch, 1 oz protein*

Progresso Healthy Favorites Minestrone: 1 cup = *1 ½ starch, 1 oz protein*

Frozen Meals

Organic Bistro's Ginger Chicken = *2 starch, 3 protein, 2 fat, 1 vegetable*

Kashi's Black Bean Mango = *2 starch, 1 fruit, 1 fat, 1 oz protein*

Trader Joe's Calabacita & Cheese Quesadilla with veggies and beans (1 quesadilla) = *2 fat, 2 starch, 1 oz protein*

Seeds of Change Lasagna Calabrese with Eggplant and Portobello Mushrooms = *1 vegetable, 2 oz protein, 2 starch, 1 fat*

Meal Bars

Kind Bar Peanut Butter & Strawberry = *2 fat, 1 starch, 1 oz protein*

18 Rabbits Nibblin' Apricot = *2 fat, 2 starch*

Larabar Apple Pie = *2 fat, 1 ½ starch*

Bumblebar Chunky Cherry = *2 fat, 1 starch*

Odwalla Chocolate Chip Peanut = *1 ½ fat, 1 oz protein, 2 starch*

Dr. Sear's Zone bars = *2 protein, 1 ½ starch, 1 ½ fat*

Kashi bars, GoLean Crisp! Chocolate Almond = *1 ½ starch, 1 oz protein, 1 fat*

Luna bar, Luna Minis = *1 starch, ½ oz protein*

Eating Out on Level 3

Restaurant meals tend to be supersized—containing far larger portions than any human being really needs. Just one fried onion appetizer served at a popular family-style restaurant, for instance, can set you back more than 1,000 calories! Another chain's shrimp and pasta dinner—something that sounds like a diet meal—contains a whopping 3,000 calories. They also tend to be loaded with fat, sugar, and other unhealthful ingredients. It's for these reasons that you will be more successful on the 2 Day Diabetes Diet if you prepare most of your own meals at home.

That said, you've got a life to live, and that includes social or business

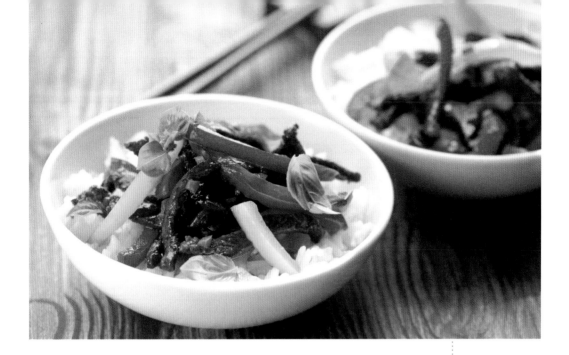

occasions that call for restaurant meals. It's best to reserve such events for Nourishment Days—or rather, since the diet schedule is up to you, it's best to schedule a Nourishment Day when there's a restaurant visit on the agenda. You may want to avoid dining out for the first several weeks on the diet, so your new eating habits are well established. After that, follow these simple tips to be sure that you don't derail your progress.

Eyeball your portions. To hold yourself to the correct portions, use the following rules of thumb.

- 3 ounces of protein = a deck of cards
- 1 cup = one tennis ball
- ¼ cup = one golf ball
- 2 tablespoons = one Ping-Pong ball
- 1 teaspoon = your thumb tip

Don't go out hungry! Eat the day's snack before going out to eat to avoid excess hunger and overeating.

Plan ahead. If possible, look at the menu in advance so you know you'll be able to find choices that fit the meal plan. You can access many restaurant menus online, and many even post the nutritional content of their menu options. Choose lower-fat menu options such as grilled or steamed fish, meats, vegetables, and salads with low-fat dressings.

Share with a friend. Restaurants tend to give us more food than we need. Share your meal with a friend, or tell the server to put half the entrée in a doggie bag before he or she brings it to the table. Or, ask for a take-home box before your meal is served. When your meal comes out, place half of your meal in the box before eating. This way you can better control your portion at the meal and not be tempted to overindulge.

Don't be afraid to substitute. Many restaurants will let you order a baked potato instead of French fries or steamed vegetables over pasta.

Avoid hidden fats. Cream sauces, butter, oils, and salad dressings add lots of fat and calories to your meal. Ask for your meal to be prepared without these fats, or order them on the side so you can control the amount you consume.

Avoid overeating by slowing down! Your brain takes 20 minutes to recognize that your stomach is full. Slow down when eating, sip on a calorie-free beverage, talk to friends, and above all, eat mindfully by paying attention to the flavor, texture, and other sensations of every bite.

Avoid alcohol. Alcohol not only can increase your appetite, it can lower your willpower when you're selecting menu items, making it more likely that you'll overindulge. Plus many mixed drinks contain enough calories to count as an entire meal. If you do drink alcoholic beverages when eating out, limit yourself to one, save it for the end of the meal, and count it as one of your treats for the week.

Watch out for high-calorie beverages. In addition to alcohol, soft drinks, sweet juices, sweetened iced tea, specialty coffee drinks, and especially milk shakes are packed full of empty calories that can elevate blood sugar and slow weight loss. Stick to water, seltzer, coffee, or tea that is either unsweetened or sweetened with a no-calorie sweetener.

Know what to watch for. Although your favorite restaurant may not post the nutritional content of the food it serves, you can make healthy choices if you do a bit of detective work. The descriptive words used to describe menu items can tell you if they have been prepared using a low-fat cooking method—or lots of added fat and calories.

Best Choices	Worst Choices
Blackened	Breaded
Braised	Buttered or butter sauce (also
Broiled	beurre, which means "butter"
Cooked in broth	in French)
Cooked in its own juice (also	Creamy/Cream sauce
known as au jus)	Crispy
Grilled	Deep fried
Poached	Fried
Roasted	Gratin
Steamed	Pan roasted
	Sautéed
	Sweet and sour
	Tempura

Special Advice for Specific Cuisines

Use these additional pointers based on the type of cuisine that will be offered where you are dining.

Fast-Food Restaurant Tips

Salads can be a healthy choice, but you have to watch what comes on them. Some salads can have more fat and calories than burgers! Choose a salad made of mixed vegetables and topped with a lean, grilled protein such as grilled chicken. Avoid added cheeses and croutons, and always ask for your dressing on the side. If adding nuts or fruit to a salad, make sure you watch the portion size and remember that this counts towards your fat and fruit servings in your meal plan.

- If choosing a sandwich, choose one made with lean protein and cooked in a low-fat method, such as a grilled instead of "crispy" or fried sandwich. If possible, order your sandwich on whole-grain bread and top it with vegetables.
- Watch out for fish. Although it sounds like a healthy option, fast-food fish is mostly fried and very high in fat and calories. If available, grilled or broiled fish is a healthy option.
- If you are craving a burger, select a small, single burger (the size of a hockey puck = 3 ounces of meat). Avoid added cheeses, sauces, and mayo. If adding ketchup or barbeque sauce, limit your serving to 1 tablespoon, as these contain a large amount of sugar.
- Chili can be a healthy option—just watch the portion. Stick to 1 cup and order a small side salad to help keep you full.
- If choosing tacos, select a soft taco (crispy tacos are fried) filled with lean protein (grilled chicken or grilled fish—watch out since the fish in fish tacos is often fried!) and vegetables.
- If choosing a sub, select the smallest size (usually 6 inches) and fill it with lean protein and vegetables. Choose the whole-grain sub roll whenever possible. For condiments, use vinegar with just a splash of oil for seasoning.
- If choosing pizza, choose a very thin-crust pizza made with whole-grain flour and topped with vegetables instead of meat.

Family Restaurant Tips

- Salads can be a great choice at these restaurants as long as you stick to a few rules. Always ask for dressing on the side and, instead of pouring it on your salad, dip each bite into the dressing to help you use less. Top your salad with lean grilled or steamed protein. Avoid added cheeses, croutons, bacon bits, crispy noodles, or nuts and fruit.
- If choosing an appetizer, choose a lean protein without additional fats such as a shrimp cocktail (just keep the cocktail sauce to 1 tablespoon) or steamed clams (avoid dipping them in butter; use lemon juice instead).

- Soups can be a great option as well, as long as they are low in fat. Minestrone soup is a great option, and so is French onion soup without the cheese and bread (just ask your server to have it prepared this way).
- Always choose lean proteins for entrées. Look for the words grilled, boiled, steamed, and broiled instead of breaded, crispy, batter dipped, pan fried, or sautéed to reduce the fat and calories of your meal.
- A vegetarian entrée such as a vegetable burger is also a low-fat protein option. Ask your server, however, how it is prepared. Avoid veggie burgers that are fried and request that yours be grilled instead. If it does come on a bun, request a whole-grain option or—even better—ask for your burger to come on a bed of fresh greens without the bun.
- If choosing a starchy side, select a plain baked potato or sweet potato (with any butter or sour cream served on the side), brown or wild rice, or a whole grain such as barley or quinoa rather than refined starches such as white pasta and white rice. Make sure to watch the portion size of your side. One-third cup to ½ cup is 1 serving for most starches.
- Avoid toppings such as creamy sauces, gravies, butter, or sour cream or food prepared au gratin, as they add significant fat and calories.

Some salads can have more fat and calories than burgers!

Italian Restaurant Tips

- Select dishes made with tomato-based sauces such as marinara, Neapolitan, cacciatore, and primavera. Lemon-based sauces such as piccata and white wine sauces are also lower fat and calorie options.
- Broiled, grilled, or steamed seafood or poultry with a side of steamed vegetables instead of pasta would be a great entrée choice. If your entrée comes over pasta, ask for it to be served over a bed of fresh greens without the pasta or with the pasta on the side.
- Try starting your meal with a garden salad (dressing on the side)

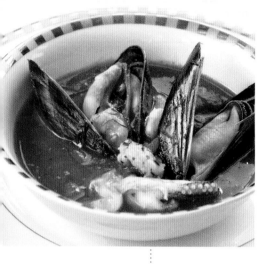

or a broth-based soup such as minestrone, eggplant, or mushroom soup to help you feel satisfied and eat a smaller portion of your entrée. A small salad and soup can also make a great meal.

▶ Avoid pasta-based dishes, as they are very high in carbohydrates and are typically made from refined carbohydrates, such as white pasta. If possible, order whole-grain pasta when available. If you do enjoy pasta, order it as a side dish rather than an entrée.

▶ For an appetizer, try a vegetable antipasto or fresh mozzarella and tomato over fried options. Roasted red peppers, grilled calamari (instead of the fried), and fresh bruschetta on whole-grain toast (if available) are also healthy options. Cioppino (a seafood stew) can also be a great appetizer or even a whole meal.

Asian Restaurant Tips

▶ Choose lean protein options such as fish and chicken over beef, pork, and duck.

▶ Ask for brown rice instead of white rice (but remember that ⅓ cup of cooked rice is equal to 1 starch serving)

▶ Look for entrées that are boiled, broiled, or steamed and include only lean protein and vegetables. For instance, try ordering steamed chicken or beef and broccoli and ask for the sauce on the side. Another option is shrimp with lobster sauce, which is made using a light wine sauce along with mushrooms, scallions, and egg.

▶ Broth-based soups are low in calories and typically lower in carbohydrates. Try miso soup, egg drop soup, sumashi soup, Thai tom yum soup (vegetarian or with fish), and canh chay soup.

▶ If ordering a tofu dish, ask for it to be prepared lightly stir-fried instead of fried.

▶ If choosing sushi, choose rolls made without rice and wrapped in seaweed (nori) or cucumber.

Mexican Restaurant Tips

- One of the biggest culprits of excess fat and calories at Mexican restaurants is cheese. Ask for dishes to be prepared without cheese or ask your server to go very light on the cheese if it is included in your entrée. The best choice would be to ask for cheese on the side (if low-fat cheese is available, request this) and sprinkle only a very small amount (¼ cup or less) on your food.

- For tacos, select soft tacos over hard tacos, as these are fried. Fill your taco with grilled chicken, fish, or shrimp, not fried, or a lean cut of beef (flank, sirloin, etc). Soft vegetarian tacos made with baked instead of refried beans are also a good option.

- Other good options include grilled or broiled seafood or poultry with a side of vegetables and baked beans, pollo picado without rice and with a side of vegetables, and chicken enchiladas prepared without cheese and sour cream (you can ask for them on the side instead).

- Traditional Mexican toppings and sides can pack on the calories and fat. Ask instead for toppings such as salsa, lime juice, and fresh guacamole (when it is made solely from avocado and seasonings). If available, low-fat sour cream would also be a healthier option. Instead of refried beans, which are fried in lard, request steamed or grilled vegetables, black beans (serving size = ½ cup), or brown rice (serving size = ⅓ cup).

- Fajitas can be a healthy option, but watch how they are prepared. Many times the vegetables and meat are sautéed in large amounts of oil. Ask for your meat and vegetables to be grilled or lightly stir-fried instead. Avoid the tortillas, cheese, and sour cream and instead place your fajita ingredients over a bed of lettuce and eat them with salsa. If you would like your fajita in a tortilla, stick to just one or two small tortillas and choose corn and whole-wheat over white flour.

- Salads can be a healthy choice at Mexican restaurants, but avoid salads that come in a fried tortilla bowl or are topped

> One of the biggest culprits of excess fat and calories is cheese.

with fried tortilla strips. Also, ask for a salad without cheese and with the dressing on the side. If your salad comes with a protein, make sure it is a lean option such as fish or chicken that has been grilled, broiled, or steamed.

▶ Try black bean soup in place of fried chips for a healthier appetizer option.

Mediterranean Restaurant Tips

▶ Salads can be loaded with high-calorie ingredients. Ask for a salad that mainly consists of leafy greens and vegetables. Ask your server to go very light on the feta or for it to be placed on the side so you can sprinkle a small amount (¼ cup or less) on your salad yourself. Have your salad topped with a lean protein choice (grilled/broiled/steamed chicken, fish, or very lean beef such as flank steak). And always have your dressing brought out on the side. Olives are fine to eat in your salad. Just remember that eight to ten olives equal 1 fat serving.

▶ If ordering kabobs or souvlakis, choose lean chicken over beef or lamb.

▶ If your meal comes with a side of rice, ask for brown or wild rice instead of white rice and watch your portion. One-third cup of rice equals 1 starch serving.

▶ If you enjoy soup, try kakavia or yogurt and cucumber soup.

▶ Sides such as rice or Greek potatoes can add many carbohydrates and calories to your meal. Instead, ask to substitute steamed vegetables or a side salad (with dressing on the side).

▶ Instead of a traditional gyro, ask for the gyro filling to be served over salad with the dressing on the side, and skip the bread and mayo altogether. Also, make sure to choose a gyro made with lean protein, like chicken breast, in place of higher-fat protein options.

THE 2 DAY WAY
Nancy Taylor

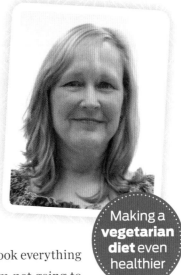

Making a **vegetarian diet** even healthier

Talk about your snow emergencies—and the need to be flexible. In just her second week on the 2 Day Diabetes Diet, publishing executive and 2 Day test panelist Nancy Taylor, 49, was trapped in a car during a commute slowed to a crawl due to an unexpected snowstorm. "It took us 6 endless hours to get home from work," she says, "and all of us in the car were dying of hunger. Next thing I know, someone starts passing out pieces of a candy bar—a candy bar! It took everything I had, but I said, nope, I'm not doing it. I've come this far, I'm not going to lose it now." Good thing it wasn't a Power Burn Day!

And she didn't. What the upstate New Yorker did lose was 10 pounds and nearly 4 inches from her waist after just 6 weeks on the 2 Day Diabetes Diet. "I was very pleasantly surprised by how tasty the food is and how easy it was for me to adapt to eating healthier," says Nancy. A breast cancer survivor, Nancy was already keenly aware of the importance of a good diet. In fact, she had become a vegetarian in part for the health benefits, but realized that it wasn't enough to ward off the risks of other diseases.

She noticed results immediately. "Within a week, my energy level was higher," she says, "and my cravings for sweets had really subsided." Which makes resisting a delectable chunk of chocolate in the middle of a snowstorm a lot easier.

The key to the 2 Day, Nancy's way:

- ▶ **She drank at least a gallon of water a day.** "The first few Power Burn Days were tough for me," says Nancy. "But I made sure to drink plenty of water, which took the edge off my hunger."
- ▶ **She kept a detailed shopping list.** "A good shopping plan is key," says Nancy, "especially in the beginning, when you have to stock your kitchen with the 2 Day foods you'll be eating.
- ▶ **She did the diet with two coworkers.** "We compared notes," says Nancy. "Did you like the fish? What veggies did you use? And as the weeks passed, we also shared our successes. What makes a success better? Getting to report it to your friends."

CHAPTER 9

The 2 Day Diabetes Diet Recipes

Enjoy almost 70 simple, scrumptious, diabetes-friendly recipes, from grab-and-go breakfasts to hearty entreés to decadent desserts.

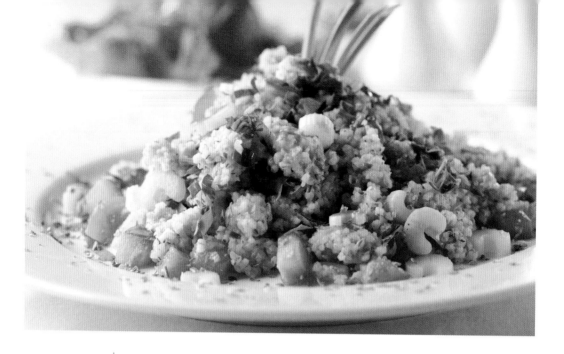

If you want to confuse your friends, tell them you're starting a new diet. Then invite them over for dinner on a Nourishment Day. After enjoying a Curried Chicken Dinner (page 205), some Zippy Shrimp (page 218), or Couscous Stuffed Peppers (page 227), your guests will be wondering why you eat better on your new diet than they do on their so-called "normal" meal plan. And there's a reason: The meals, recipes, and food choices in the 2 Day Diabetes Diet are designed to be so flavorful and satisfying that, on some Nourishment Days, you'll probably forget you're even on a diet.

In the following pages, you'll find dozens of mouthwatering recipes. They either correspond to recommended meals in Levels 1 and 2 of the 2 Day Diabetes Diet or they can be used to create your own Level 3 meals. If you are using a recipe as part of Level 1 or 2 of the plan, all of the number crunching has been done for you within the menus and food lists in Chapters 6 and 7. Just follow the suggestions listed in those chapters for side dishes.

If you are using Level 3 of the plan, then check the nutrition info that accompanies each recipe. In addition to the standard list of calories, carbohydrates, protein, fats, and other nutrients you get per serving of that recipe, you'll see that we've listed the 2 Day Diabetes Diet exchanges of starch, dairy, and other 2 Day Diabetes Diet food groups—so you can match those up with your daily goals. (If you are used to using the diabetes exchanges, created by the American Diabetes Association and American Diabetic Association, you'll see that these match up pretty closely, but they are designed specifically for this plan, so you may notice some variations.)

No matter what level of the plan you are following, keep the following pointers in mind.

- We've tried to feature superfoods and super spices and seasonings whenever possible. That said, not all recipes include these important foods. For best results on the 2 Day Diabetes Diet, try to consume these superfoods and super spices and seasonings at least three times a week.
- Although some recipes include artificial sweeteners, you don't want to develop a reliance on these, for reasons we've already mentioned. Try not to sweeten recipes even more by adding more sweetener than a recipe calls for, and, for best results, limit yourself to only one food or recipe a day that contains artificial sweeteners.
- To convert a meat recipe into a vegetarian recipe, consult the 2 Day Diabetes Diet Formula on page 146. Swap in 1 serving of plant-based protein for 1 serving of animal protein.
- If you don't do dairy, just swap in a nondairy milk (almond, coconut, soy) for cow's milk. Note that almond milk is lower in protein than cow's milk and other milk substitutes. If you use this variety, add 1 extra ounce of protein per cup.
- It's okay to make other substitutions as needed—for instance, to sub in collards for spinach and strawberries for blueberries. Just try to swap like foods. Don't, for instance, swap a fruit for a vegetable or a starchy vegetable for a nonstarchy vegetable.

The recipes are so flavorful and satisfying, you'll probably forget you're on a diet.

Spices are unlimited on the plan, so feel free to add more flavor as needed. However, don't add salt, as it might contribute to high blood pressure. Seventy percent of people with diabetes have high blood pressure, probably because high blood sugar can irritate the linings of your arteries, hardening them. This makes it tougher for your heart to pump blood, raising the pressure inside your arteries and causing hypertension. In addition to being more prone to high blood pressure, you are probably also salt sensitive. That means that your body retains more water in an attempt to flush salt, raising your blood pressure as a result.

The recipes of the 2 Day Diabetes Diet are naturally low in sodium. They are brimming with fresh produce, whole grains, and unprocessed foods that are naturally low in sodium. And these foods are also packed with important nutrients—like potassium, magnesium, and calcium—that work hard to keep your blood pressure levels healthy. Stick to just 2,300 milligrams or less of sodium a day if you are healthy or prone to developing diabetes. That's the amount in 1 teaspoon of salt. If you have diabetes plus hypertension (high blood pressure), you should aim for 1,500 milligrams or less daily.

FAQ: WHAT ARE SOME EASY WAYS TO CONSUME LESS SODIUM?

Choosing fresh and less-processed foods is a great way to reduce your sodium intake dramatically. Some examples:

CHOOSING THIS . . .	INSTEAD OF THAT . . .	SAVES THIS MUCH SODIUM
1 fresh tomato slice	1 tablespoon of ketchup on your burger	166 mg
Homemade salad dressing	Bottled salad dressing	505 mg per 2 tablespoons
Baby carrots	Pretzels (1 oz)	380 mg
Brown rice	Packaged, seasoned rice	950 mg per serving
Dry-roasted almonds	Salted almonds	96 mg per 1 oz serving

Depending on what brands of foods you choose, you may sometimes find measurements listed in metrics, so we've included a conversion chart here to make it easier for you to follow the 2 Day Diabetes Diet recipes no matter where you are!

Conversion Chart

ABBREVIATIONS

C	Celsius
cm	centimeter
F	Fahrenheit
fl oz	fluid ounce
ft	foot
g	gram
gal	gallon
in.	inch
kg	kilogram
L	liter
lb	pound
m	meter
mL	milliliter
mm	millimeter
oz	ounce
qt	quart
tbsp	tablespoon
tsp	teaspoon

TEASPOONS

⅛ tsp	0.5 mL
¼ tsp	1 mL
½ tsp	2 mL
¾ tsp	4 mL
1 tsp	5 mL
1½ tsp	7 mL
2 tsp	10 mL

TABLESPOONS

1 tbsp	15 mL
1½ tbsp	20 mL
2 tbsp	30 mL
3 tbsp	45 mL
4 tbsp	60 mL
5 tbsp	75 mL
6 tbsp	90 mL
8 tbsp	125 mL

WEIGHTS

1 oz	30 g
2 oz	60 g
3 oz	90 g
4 oz	125 g
5 oz	150 g
6 oz	175 g
8 oz	250 g
10 oz	300 g
12 oz	375 g
16 oz	500 g
32 oz	1 kg
¼ lb	125 g
½ lb	250 g
⅔ lb	300 g
¾ lb	375 g
1 lb	500 g
2 lb	1 kg
3 lb	1.5 kg

LENGTHS

¼ in.	5 mm
½ in.	1 cm
1 in.	2.5 cm
2 in.	5 cm
6 in.	15 cm
1 ft	30 cm

VOLUME

1 fl oz	30 mL
2 fl oz	50 mL
5 fl oz	150 mL
10 fl oz	300 mL
1 pint	500 mL
1 qt	1 L
1 gal	4 L
¼ cup	60 mL
⅓ cup	75 mL
½ cup	125 mL
⅔ cup	150 mL
¾ cup	175 mL
1 cup	250 mL
1¼ cups	300 mL
1½ cups	375 mL
2 cups	500 mL
4 cups	1 L
6 cups	1.5 L

OVEN TEMPERATURES

°F	°C
175°F	80°C
200°F	95°C
225°F	110°C
250°F	120°C
275°F	140°C
300°F	150°C
325°F	160°C
350°F	180°C
375°F	190°C
400°F	200°C
425°F	220°C
450°F	230°C
475°F	240°C
500°F	260°C

BAKING PANS

8 x 8 in.	20 x 20 cm
9 x 9 in.	22 x 22 cm
9 x 13 in.	22 x 33 cm
10 x 15 in.	25 x 38 cm
11 x 17 in.	28 x 43 cm
8 x 2 in. (round)	20 x 5 cm
9 x 2 in. (round)	22 x 5 cm
10 x 4 ½ in. (tube)	25 x 11 cm
8 x 4 x 3 in. (loaf)	20 x 10 x 7.5 cm
9 x 5 x 3 in. (loaf)	22 x 12.5 x 7.5 cm

CASSEROLE DISHES

Recipe calls for	Substitute
1 qt (4 cups)	900 mL
1 ½ qt (6 cups)	1.35 L
2–2 ½ qt (8–10 cups)	2.25 L
3 qt (12 cups)	2.7 L
4–5 qt (16–20 cups)	4.5 L

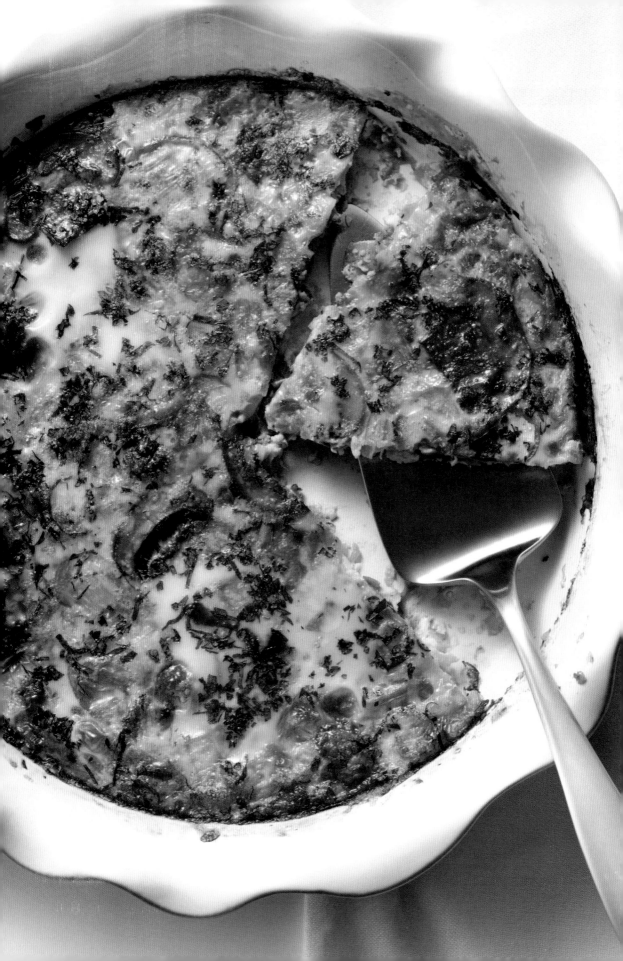

Mushroom Quiche

This simple, no-crust quiche is the perfect combination of protein and vegetables to satisfy your appetite. Make it ahead and eat it throughout the week.

Makes 4 servings

1 cup chopped onion

1 cup chopped mushrooms

1 cup liquid egg whites
(or 8 egg whites)

1. Preheat the oven to 375°F and spray an 8" square glass baking pan with nonstick cooking spray.

2. Coat a saucepan with cooking spray and place it over medium heat. Sauté the onion and mushrooms until tender.

3. Pour half of the egg whites into the prepared baking pan.

4. Evenly spread the onion and mushroom mixture on top of the egg mixture.

5. Pour the remaining egg whites on top, covering the vegetables.

6. Place the baking pan in the oven and bake for 30 minutes, or until a toothpick inserted in the center comes out clean.

PER SERVING **Nutrition info:** 50 calories, 7 g protein, 5 g carbohydrate, 0 g total fat, 0 g saturated fat, 0 mg cholesterol, 1 g fiber, 101 mg sodium

2 Day Diabetes Diet exchanges: 1 vegetable, 1 oz protein

Peanut Butter Tortilla

We're convinced that this is the simplest tortilla roll-up you'll ever make, and it's perfect for eating on the go.

Makes 1 serving

2 teaspoons natural peanut butter

1 whole-grain tortilla (6" diameter)

15 raisins

Spread the peanut butter thinly over the tortilla. Sprinkle the raisins evenly over the peanut butter. Roll up the tortilla. Serve at room temperature or microwave on high for 30 seconds and serve warm.

PER SERVING **Nutrition info:** 232 calories, 6 g protein, 36 g carbohydrate, 8 g total fat, 2 g saturated fat, 0 mg cholesterol, 1 g fiber, 196 mg sodium

2 Day Diabetes Diet exchanges: 1 fruit, 1 starch, 1 fat

Banana Toast

Elvis was on to something with his fried peanut butter and banana sandwich. This version is just as good, but without all the disease-promoting fat.

Makes 1 serving

1 slice whole-grain bread

2 teaspoons natural almond butter

½ banana, thinly sliced

Toast the bread. Spread the almond butter over the warm bread and top with the sliced banana. Serve warm.

PER SERVING **Nutrition info:** 181 calories, 5 g protein, 27 g carbohydrate, 8 g total fat, 1 g saturated fat, 0 mg cholesterol, 4 g fiber, 134 mg sodium

2 Day Diabetes Diet exchanges: 1 fruit, 1 starch, 1 fat

Multigrain Pancakes

Too often pancakes are full of refined, blood-sugar-spiking flour. This version, however, uses wheat germ and whole-grain flour to render these treats blood sugar friendly.

Makes 8 servings (2 pancakes each)

- 2 cups low-fat buttermilk
- ½ cup old-fashioned rolled oats
- ⅔ cup whole-wheat flour
- ⅔ cup all-purpose flour
- ¼ cup toasted wheat germ
- 1½ teaspoons baking powder
- ½ teaspoon baking soda
- ¼ teaspoon salt
- 1 teaspoon ground cinnamon
- 2 large eggs
- ¼ cup firmly packed brown sugar
- 1 tablespoon canola oil
- 2 teaspoons vanilla extract
- 1 cup maple syrup, warmed
- 1½ cups sliced strawberries or blueberries

1. Preheat the oven to 200°F. Mix the buttermilk and oats in a small bowl. Let stand for 15 minutes.

2. Whisk the whole-wheat flour, all-purpose flour, wheat germ, baking powder, baking soda, salt, and cinnamon in a large bowl.

3. Whisk the eggs, sugar, oil, and vanilla in a medium bowl. Add the buttermilk mixture. Add this mixture to the flour mixture and mix with a rubber spatula just until moistened.

4. Coat a large nonstick skillet with cooking spray. Heat over medium heat. Spoon about ¼ cup batter for each pancake into the skillet and cook until the bottoms are golden and small bubbles start to form on top, about 3 minutes. Flip the pancakes and cook until browned and cooked through, 1 to 2 minutes longer. (Adjust the heat as necessary for even browning.) Keep the pancakes warm in the oven while you finish cooking the remaining batter.

5. Top with maple syrup and strawberries or blueberries and serve. Wrap any leftover pancakes individually in plastic wrap and refrigerate for up to 2 days or freeze for up to 1 month. Reheat in a toaster or toaster oven.

PER SERVING **Nutrition info:** 292 calories, 8 g protein, 60 g carbohydrate, 3 g total fat, 1 g saturated fat, 56 mg cholesterol, 3 g fiber, 331 mg sodium

2 Day Diabetes Diet exchanges: 4 starch, 1 oz protein, ½ fat

Blueberry Muffins

These delicious muffins are packed full of slimming nutrition. Count the blueberries inside as one of your 3 weekly servings of superfoods.

Makes 24 muffins

1   cup bran cereal (such as All-Bran or Fiber One)

1½ cups mashed banana or unsweetened applesauce

¼   cup fat-free milk

1   cup whole-wheat flour

½   cup old-fashioned oats

1   tablespoon baking powder

½   teaspoon baking soda

1   tablespoon honey

2   tablespoons dark molasses

1   teaspoon ground cinnamon

2   egg whites or 1 whole egg or ¼ cup liquid egg substitute

⅔   cup blueberries or ¼ cup dried cranberries and ¼ cup mini chocolate chips

1. Preheat the oven to 400°F. Spray two 12-cup muffin pans with cooking spray or insert paper liners.

2. Combine the cereal, banana, and milk in a large bowl. Let stand for about 5 minutes.

3. Add the flour, oats, baking powder, baking soda, honey, molasses, cinnamon, egg whites, and blueberries and stir until combined. Spoon the batter into the pans and bake for 20 minutes.

PER MUFFIN **Nutrition info:** 60 calories, 2 g protein, 13 g carbohydrate, 0 g total fat, 0 g saturated fat, 0 mg cholesterol, 3 g fiber, 106 mg sodium

2 Day Diabetes Diet exchanges: 1 starch

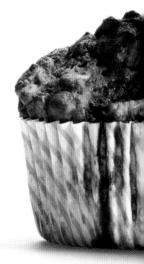

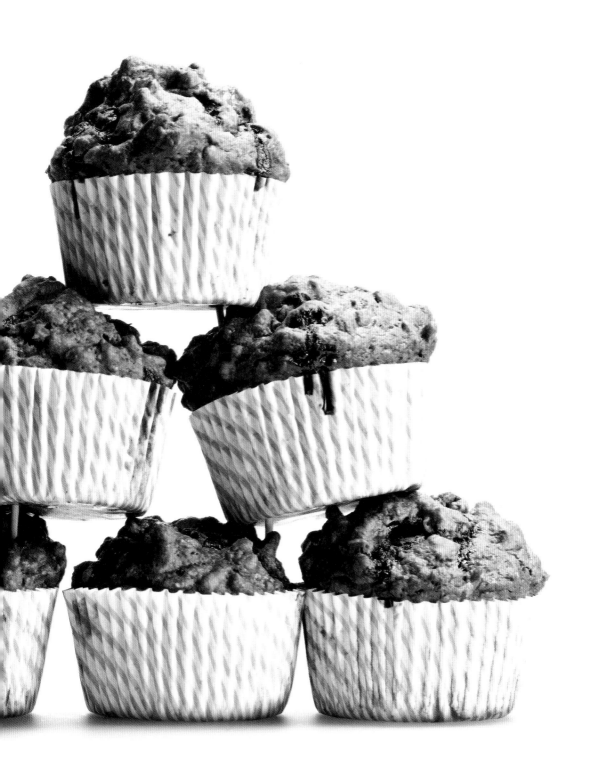

Oatmeal with Apple and Flaxseeds

If you've avoided oatmeal in the past, give this version a try. The apple and cinnamon combo is enough to turn anyone into a lover of this important superfood.

Makes 4 servings (⅔ cup each)

- 2 cups 1% milk or vanilla soy milk

- ¾ cup old-fashioned rolled oats (not quick oats)

- 1 medium apple, peeled, cored, and chopped

- ⅓ cup dried cranberries or raisins

- ½ teaspoon ground cinnamon

- ¼ cup whole flaxseeds, ground, or ⅓ cup flaxseed meal

- ¼ cup fat-free plain or vanilla yogurt

- ¼ cup maple syrup, warmed, or 2 tablespoons brown sugar

1. Combine the milk, rolled oats, apple, dried cranberries or raisins, and cinnamon in a heavy medium saucepan. Bring to a boil over medium-high heat, stirring almost constantly.

2. Reduce the heat to medium-low and cook, stirring often, for 3 to 5 minutes or until creamy and thickened.

3. Stir in the flaxseeds. Spoon the oatmeal into individual bowls and top each serving with a dollop of yogurt and a drizzle of maple syrup or bit of brown sugar. Leftovers will keep, covered, in the refrigerator for up to 2 days. Reheat in the microwave.

PER SERVING **Nutrition info:** 282 calories, 10 g protein, 47 g carbohydrate, 7 g total fat, 1 g saturated fat, 8 mg cholesterol, 6 g fiber, 84 mg sodium

2 Day Diabetes Diet exchanges: ½ fruit, 1 ½ starch, ½ dairy

Baked Apple

Why save baked apples for dessert when they make for an easy breakfast option, one that's full of appetite-suppressing pectin?

Makes 1 serving

- 1 medium apple, sliced
- 1 teaspoon grapeseed oil or olive oil
- 1 tablespoon ground cinnamon

1. Preheat the oven to 350°F (or you may use the microwave oven for this recipe). Place the apple slices in a glass bowl and top them with the oil and cinnamon.

2. Bake in the oven for 10 to 15 minutes (or microwave on high for 5 minutes).

3. Test for doneness. The apple should be tender. If still firm, bake for 3 to 5 minutes longer in the oven (or microwave 1 to 2 minutes longer). Serve warm.

PER SERVING **Nutrition info:** 121 calories, 0 g protein, 21 g carbohydrate, 5 g total fat, 1 g saturated fat, 0 mg cholesterol, 4 g fiber, 0 mg sodium

2 Day Diabetes Diet exchanges: 1 fruit, 1 fat

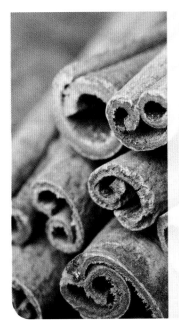

SUPERFOOD SPOTLIGHT: Cinnamon

Several studies show that this delicious spice can help reduce blood sugar. In one of them, published in the journal *Diabetes Care,* people with type 2 diabetes who'd taken 1 or more grams of cinnamon daily dropped their fasting blood sugar by a whopping 30 percent compared to people who took no cinnamon. They also reduced their triglycerides, LDL cholesterol, and total cholesterol by upwards of 25 percent.[1] At work here are two important nutrients. Cinnamon is rich in chromium, a mineral that enhances the effects of insulin. It's also loaded with polyphenols, antioxidants that gather up all the free radicals in your blood to protect you from cancer and also lower systemic inflammation, further protecting you from diabetes and heart disease. Best of all, cinnamon makes everything more delicious. Use a cinnamon stick to stir your tea, and throw it in everything you're already eating and drinking—coffee, hot tea, oatmeal, yogurt, even chili or spaghetti sauce.

Round Steak Chili

Don't let the number of ingredients fool you. This recipe is as easy as dumping everything into one pot, turning on a burner, and relaxing.

Makes 10 servings (1 cup each)

1 pound beef round steak, trimmed and cut into ½" cubes

1 large onion, chopped

2 garlic cloves, minced

1 can (46 ounces) V8 juice

1 can (28 ounces) crushed tomatoes

2 cups sliced celery

1 medium green pepper, chopped

1 bay leaf

2 tablespoons chili powder

1 teaspoon dried oregano

1 teaspoon brown sugar

½ teaspoon celery seed

½ teaspoon paprika

½ teaspoon ground mustard

½ teaspoon ground cumin

¼ teaspoon cayenne pepper

¼ teaspoon dried basil

1 can (16 ounces) kidney beans, rinsed and drained

1. In a large kettle or Dutch oven coated with nonstick cooking spray, brown the meat, onion, and garlic.

2. Add the V8, tomatoes, celery, green pepper, bay leaf, chili powder, oregano, brown sugar, celery seed, paprika, mustard, cumin, cayenne pepper, and basil. Bring to a boil. Reduce the heat and simmer, uncovered, for 3 hours.

3. Add the kidney beans and heat through. Remove the bay leaf before serving.

PER SERVING **Nutrition info:** 200 calories, 22 g protein, 22 g carbohydrate, 3 g total fat, 1 g saturated fat, 40 mg cholesterol, 7 g fiber, 240 mg sodium

2 Day Diabetes Diet exchanges: 2 vegetables, ½ starch, 3 oz protein

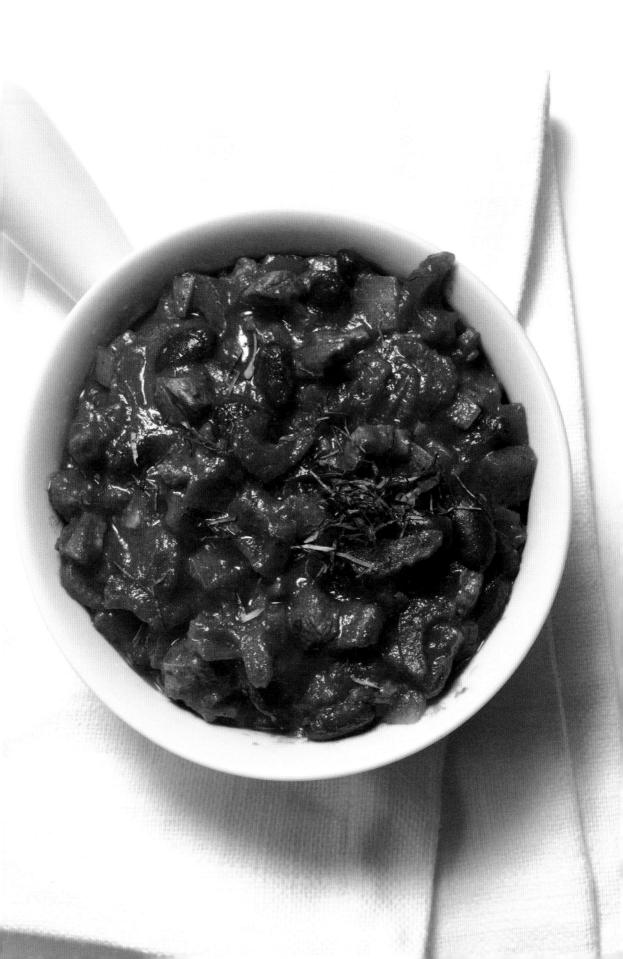

New Mexican Green Chili

Spicy foods help to fill you up on fewer calories, and they boost calorie burning, too. When cutting or seeding hot peppers, use rubber or plastic gloves to protect your hands, and avoid touching your face.

Makes 4 servings

1   tablespoon olive oil

1   pound well-trimmed pork tenderloin, cut into 1" chunks

5   scallions, thinly sliced

4   cloves garlic, minced

2   large green bell peppers, cut into ½" cubes

2   pickled jalapeño peppers, seeded and minced

2   teaspoons ground cumin

2   teaspoons ground coriander

½   teaspoon salt

1   cup water

1   can (15 ounces) garbanzo beans, rinsed and drained

½   cup chopped cilantro

1. Heat the oil in a nonstick Dutch oven over medium-high heat. Brown the pork for about 4 minutes. With a slotted spoon, transfer the pork to a plate.

2. Reduce the heat to medium. Add the scallions and garlic and cook until the scallions are tender, about 2 minutes. Stir in the bell and jalapeño peppers and cook until the bell peppers are tender, about 4 minutes.

3. Return the pork to the pan. Add the cumin, coriander, and salt. Stir. Add the water and bring to a boil. Reduce to a simmer, cover, and cook for 20 minutes.

4. Stir in the garbanzo beans. Cover and cook until the garbanzo beans are heated through, about 5 minutes. Stir in the cilantro before serving.

PER SERVING **Nutrition info:** 300 calories, 31 g protein, 24 g carbohydrate, 10 g total fat, 2 g saturated fat, 74 mg cholesterol, 7 g fiber, 565 mg sodium

2 Day Diabetes Diet exchanges: 1 vegetable, 1 starch, 5 oz protein, 1 fat

Bouillon Vegetable Soup

Make plenty of this hunger stopper ahead of time so you have it on hand during Power Burn Days. It's so satisfying that you'll have a hard time believing it contains only 80 calories per serving.

Makes 1 serving

¼ cup chopped onion

¼ cup chopped celery

¼ cup grated carrots

¼ cup diced tomatoes

1 tablespoon garlic powder

1 teaspoon onion powder

1 teaspoon ground black pepper

1 beef bouillon cube

1 cup hot water

1. In a Dutch oven sprayed with nonstick cooking spray over medium heat, cook the onions, celery, and carrots for 5 minutes, or until tender.

2. Add the tomatoes, garlic powder, onion powder, and pepper and cook for 2 minutes longer.

3. In a small bowl or cup, add the bouillon cube to the water. Once it has dissolved, add it to the vegetables. Allow the soup to simmer over medium heat for 10 minutes. Serve warm.

PER SERVING **Nutrition info:** 80 calories, 3 g protein, 18 g carbohydrate, 0.5 g total fat, 0 g saturated fat, 0 mg cholesterol, 3 g fiber, 74 mg sodium

2 Day Diabetes Diet exchanges: 1 vegetable, 8 oz bouillon

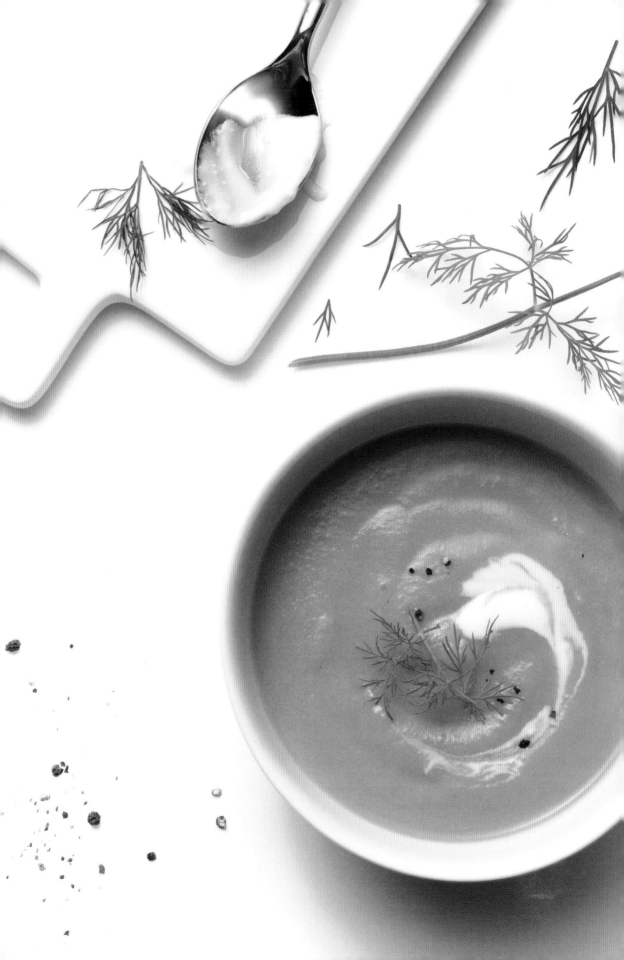

Carrot Soup with Dill

You can consume this sweet and savory soup either hot or chilled, making it a versatile option for any season.

Makes 4 servings

1 tablespoon vegetable oil

1 onion, coarsely chopped

1 clove garlic, minced

2 cans (14 ½ ounces each) reduced-sodium, fat-free chicken broth

1 ¼ pounds carrots, peeled and coarsely chopped (4 cups)

½ teaspoon dried thyme, crumbled

¼ teaspoon salt

¼ teaspoon white pepper

¼ cup low-fat plain yogurt

1 tablespoon finely chopped dill

1. In a medium saucepan over medium heat, heat the oil. Add the onion and garlic. Sauté 5 minutes, or until softened. Add the broth, carrots, and thyme. Simmer, uncovered, until the vegetables are very tender, about 40 minutes.

2. In batches, puree the soup in a blender. Add the salt and pepper. To serve hot, ladle into bowls and garnish each bowl with the yogurt and dill. To serve cold, remove from the heat and let cool to room temperature. Cover and refrigerate until cold. Garnish just before serving.

PER SERVING **Nutrition info:** 135 calories, 6 g protein, 20 g carbohydrate, 4 g total fat, 0 g saturated fat, 1 mg cholesterol, 5 g fiber, 773 mg sodium

2 Day Diabetes Diet exchanges: 1 vegetable, 1 fat, 8 oz bouillon

Summer Garden Soup

As its name implies, this incredibly filling soup makes great use of summer vegetables that are easy to grow in a home garden.

Makes 6 servings

2	teaspoons olive oil
1	medium onion, finely chopped
1	large stalk celery, finely chopped
2	teaspoons peeled, finely chopped fresh ginger
¼	pound green beans, cut into 1 ½" pieces
2	medium potatoes, unpeeled and cut into ½" cubes
1	large carrot, peeled and cut into ½" cubes
1	medium yellow summer squash, quartered lengthwise, seeded, and cut into ½" cubes
8	cups water
1	bay leaf
¾	teaspoon salt
¾	cup fresh or frozen green peas
2	plum tomatoes, seeded and coarsely chopped
2	tablespoons finely chopped fresh basil leaves
1½	teaspoons finely chopped fresh thyme leaves

1. In a large pot over medium heat, heat the oil. Sauté the onion, celery, and ginger for about 10 minutes, or until very tender. Add the green beans, potatoes, carrot, squash, water, bay leaf, and salt. Simmer, covered, for 20 minutes.

2. Uncover the soup. Simmer for 15 minutes longer. During the last 5 minutes, add the peas, tomatoes, basil, and thyme. Remove the bay leaf before serving.

PER SERVING **Nutrition info:** 88 calories, 3 g protein, 17 g carbohydrate, 2 g total fat, 0 g saturated fat, 0 mg cholesterol, 4 g fiber, 307 mg sodium

2 Day Diabetes Diet exchanges: 1 vegetable, 1 starch

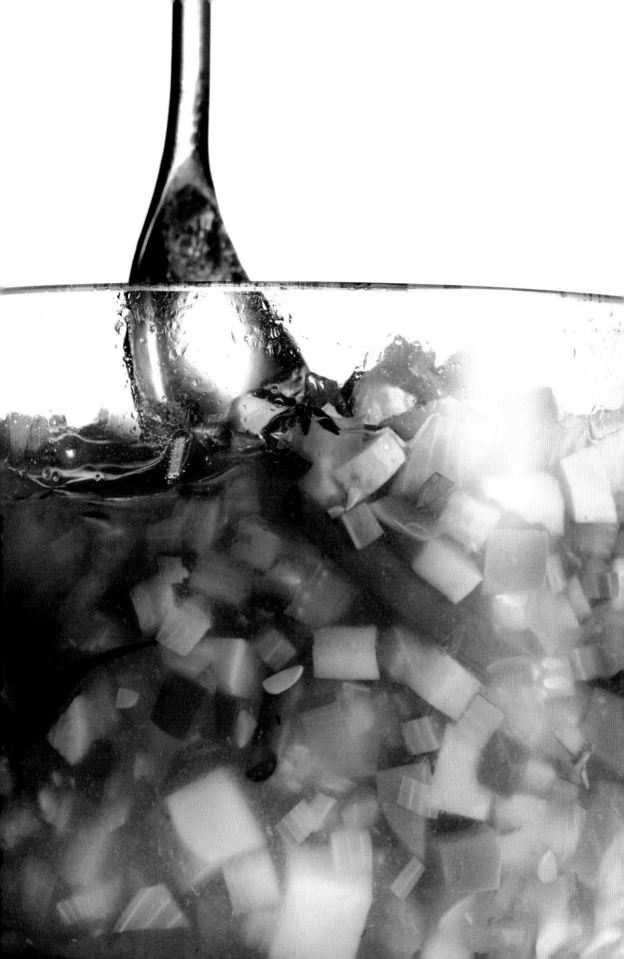

Creamy Greens Soup

Greens not only help prevent diabetes, they also protect against heart disease and cancer, and this recipe is chock-full of them.

Makes 8 servings

- 2 teaspoons olive oil
- 2 leeks, pale green and white parts only, rinsed and coarsely chopped
- 1 medium onion, coarsely chopped
- 2 cloves garlic, minced
- 1 small bunch collard greens, stemmed and coarsely chopped
- 1 small bunch Swiss chard, stemmed and coarsely chopped
- 2 medium Yukon Gold or all-purpose potatoes, unpeeled and coarsely chopped
- 1 carrot, peeled and coarsely chopped
- 2 cans (14 ½ ounces each) reduced-sodium, fat-free chicken broth
- 4 cups water
- 1 teaspoon salt
- ½ cup half-and-half

1. In a large pot over medium heat, heat oil. Add the leeks and onion. Sauté until softened, about 5 minutes. Add the garlic and sauté 2 minutes longer. Add the collard greens, Swiss chard, potatoes, and carrot. Stir in the broth, water, and salt. Simmer, partially covered, for 50 minutes.

2. In a blender or food processor, puree the soup in small batches. Return to the pot. Stir in the half-and-half. Heat just until warmed through.

PER SERVING Nutrition info: 124 calories, 5 g protein, 20 g carbohydrate, 4 g total fat, 2 g saturated fat, 7 mg cholesterol, 5 g fiber, 459 mg sodium

2 Day Diabetes Diet exchanges: ½ vegetable, ½ starch, 1 fat, 4 oz bouillon

SUPERFOOD SPOTLIGHT: Collard Greens

Dark green leafy vegetables like collard greens are tops for vitamin C, which helps lower cortisol in the body, consequently reducing inflammation as well. Collard greens (and other cruciferous veggies like kale and Brussels sprouts) are also a good source of alpha-lipoic acid (ALA), a micronutrient that also helps the body deal with stress. When scientists at the Linus Pauling Institute at Oregon State University gave aging rats ALA, they found that their bodies created their own antioxidants, making them better able to resist toxins in the environment, and reduce inflammation.[2] Good news for people with diabetes: ALA also helps reduces blood sugar and can help to strengthen the nerves damaged by diabetic neuropathy. Just be careful not to overcook it, which creates that stinky sulfur smell. Just 5 minutes of steaming, and you're done!

Winter Vegetable Soup

This veggie-packed soup will stick to your ribs and warm you up, but, at only 50 calories per serving, it definitely won't stick to your fat cells.

Makes 14 servings

2 cans (16 ounces each) whole tomatoes

1 can (16 ounces) tomato sauce

1 quart water

4 beef bouillon cubes

1 to 2 cloves garlic, chopped

1 large turnip, coarsely chopped

1 green bell pepper, coarsely chopped

½ stalk celery, coarsely chopped

1 large onion, coarsely chopped

1 small zucchini, coarsely chopped

2 large carrots, coarsely chopped

1 small head cabbage, shredded

8 ounces fresh or frozen green beans

1 cup frozen chopped spinach, thawed

1 teaspoon dried thyme

1 teaspoon dried oregano

1 bay leaf

   Salt and freshly ground black pepper to taste

1. Combine the tomatoes, tomato sauce, water, bouillon, and garlic in a large soup pot. Add the turnip, bell pepper, celery, onion, zucchini, and carrots to the pot.

2. Bring to a boil, reduce heat and simmer for at least 1 hour, or until the vegetables are somewhat softened but still firm. Stir in the cabbage, beans, spinach, thyme, oregano, bay leaf, salt, and pepper.

3. Simmer until the vegetables are cooked through but still firm. Discard the bay leaf before serving.

PER SERVING **Nutrition info:** 50 calories, 3 g protein, 11 g carbohydrate, 0 g total fat, 0 g saturated fat, 0 mg cholesterol, 3 g fiber, 625 mg sodium

2 Day Diabetes Diet exchanges: 1 ½ vegetable, 8 oz bouillon

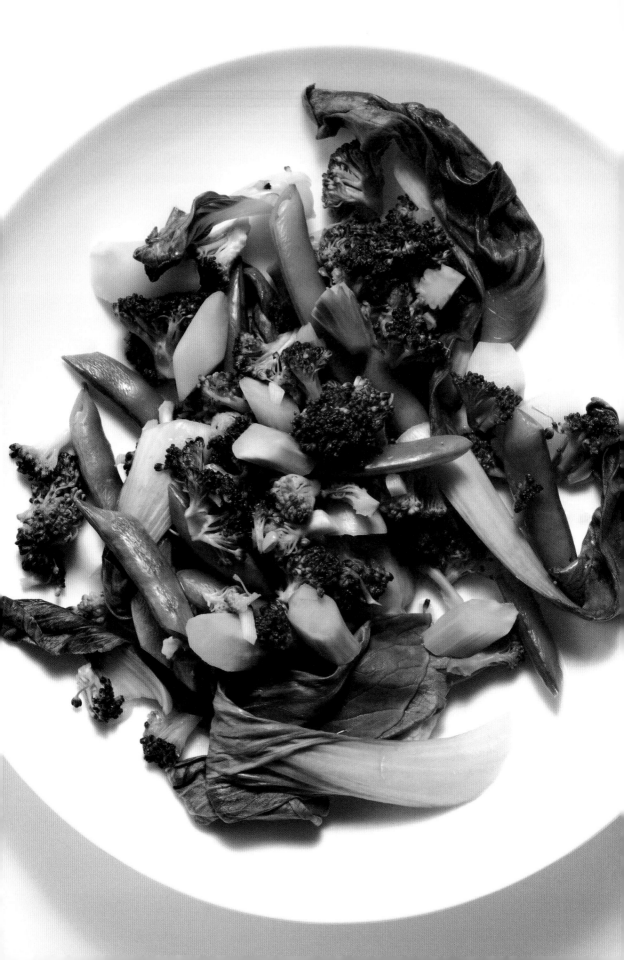

Warm Green Vegetable Salad

This Asian-themed salad is served warm, making it the perfect fiber-packed side dish for any meal of your choice.

Makes 4 servings

½ pound broccoli, cut into small florets, stalk peeled and cut diagonally into ½" slices

½ pound small bok choy or other Chinese greens, trimmed and stem sliced

4 scallions, cut diagonally into thin slices

¼ pound sugar snaps, trimmed

1 small clove garlic, crushed

1 teaspoon finely grated peeled fresh ginger

1 teaspoon dark brown sugar

1 tablespoon Thai fish sauce

1. Fill a steamer pot with water to just below the basket. Bring the water to a boil.

2. In a large bowl, combine the broccoli, bok choy, scallions, and sugar snaps. Add the garlic and ginger and toss well. Transfer to the steamer basket, cover, and steam for 3 to 4 minutes, or until the vegetables are tender-crisp.

3. In a small cup, combine the sugar and fish sauce, stirring until the sugar dissolves. Arrange the vegetables in a serving dish and drizzle with this dressing. Serve hot, or let cool and then refrigerate until 10 minutes before serving.

PER SERVING **Nutrition info:** 50 calories, 4 g protein, 9 g carbohydrate, 0 g total fat, 0 g saturated fat, 0 mg cholesterol, 3 g fiber, 400 mg sodium

2 Day Diabetes Diet exchanges: 1 vegetable

Southwestern Black Bean Salad

This salad can be tossed together quickly before a summer get-together, allowing you to stay true to the 2 Day Diabetes Diet at cookouts, covered dish events, and much more.

Makes 10 servings

- 2 cans (16 ounces each) black beans, drained and rinsed
- 1 can (16 ounces) whole kernel corn, drained
- 2 teaspoons minced garlic
- 1 medium green or red bell pepper, chopped
- ½ cup minced onion
- ½ cup lime juice
- 2 teaspoons dried cumin
- 2 teaspoons dried oregano
- 2 tablespoons chopped parsley
- 1 teaspoon crushed red pepper (optional)
- ½ cup cooked barley (optional)

1. Stir together the beans, corn, garlic, bell pepper, onion, lime juice, cumin, oregano, parsley, red pepper (if desired), and barley (if desired) in a large bowl.

2. Mix well and serve chilled or heated.

PER SERVING **Nutrition info:** 120 calories, 7 g protein, 23 g carbohydrate, 0 g total fat, 0 g saturated fat, 0 mg cholesterol, 7 g fiber, 135 mg sodium

2 Day Diabetes Diet exchanges: 1 starch, 1 oz protein

Asian Salad with Creamy Ginger Dressing

If you don't do dairy, then you'll love this creamy dressing made from tofu. To make ginger juice, put a ½-inch piece of fresh ginger through a garlic press or grate the ginger and press out the juice with a spoon; discard the pulp.

Makes 4 servings

For the dressing:

- 4 ounces soft tofu
- ¼ cup water
- 1 tablespoon reduced-sodium soy sauce
- 1 clove garlic, crushed
- 2 teaspoons rice vinegar
- ½ teaspoon ginger juice
- ¼ teaspoon sugar

For the salad:

- 1 small head romaine lettuce or 6 ounces spinach, cut into 1"-wide ribbons (6 cups)
- 2 medium carrots, shredded (1 ½ cups)
- 4 radishes, thinly sliced (⅓ cup)

1. To prepare the dressing: In a food processor or blender, whirl the tofu, water, soy sauce, garlic, vinegar, ginger juice, and sugar for 1 minute or until smooth.

2. To prepare the salad: In a large salad bowl, place the lettuce, carrots, and radishes. Pour the dressing over the vegetables and toss until coated.

PER SERVING **Nutrition info:** 55 calories, 4 g protein, 8 g carbohydrate, 1 g total fat, 0 g saturated fat, 0 mg cholesterol, 3 g fiber, 143 mg sodium

2 Day Diabetes Diet exchanges: 2 vegetable, 1 oz protein

Picnic Lemon-Rice Salad

This cool rice salad is the perfect 2 Day Diabetes Diet option for summer cookouts. Easy to tote and with a fresh lemon taste, it's a light dish that goes with any grilled seafood or poultry.

Makes 2 servings

2 cups cooked brown rice

1 cup diced, seeded tomato

1 cup frozen green peas, thawed

1 carrot, diced

2 scallions, minced

¼ cup fresh parsley, minced

3 tablespoons fat-free mayonnaise

1 tablespoon lemon juice

½ teaspoon lemon zest

Salt and ground black pepper, to taste

In a large bowl, combine the rice with the tomato, peas, carrot, scallions, and parsley. In a separate bowl, whisk together the mayonnaise, lemon juice, lemon zest, and salt and pepper. Add to the rice salad and toss well.

PER SERVING **Nutrition info:** 329 calories, 10 g protein, 67 g carbohydrate, 2 g total fat, 0 g saturated fat, 0 mg cholesterol, 10 g fiber, 423 mg sodium

2 Day Diabetes Diet exchanges: 1 vegetable, 4 starch

Grilled Vegetable Salad

This summer salad is great for those days when it's too hot to cook indoors. Just throw all your ingredients onto the grill and enjoy.

Makes 6 servings

- 1 small eggplant (¾ pound), cut lengthwise into ½" slices
- 1 small bulb fennel (6 ounces), trimmed and cut lengthwise into ½" slices
- 1 medium yellow summer squash, cut lengthwise into ½" slices
- 1 medium zucchini, cut lengthwise into ½" slices
- ½ teaspoon salt, divided
- 1 small red bell pepper, halved lengthwise and seeded
- 3 plum tomatoes, halved lengthwise and seeded
- 2 tablespoons olive oil
- 2 cloves garlic, minced
- 1 teaspoon finely chopped fresh marjoram or ½ teaspoon dried, crumbled
- 1½ tablespoons balsamic vinegar

1. Preheat the grill to medium-high. Sprinkle the eggplant, fennel, squash, and zucchini slices with ¼ teaspoon of the salt and spray them generously with cooking spray.

2. Grill the pepper, skin side down, until blackened and blistered, 3 to 4 minutes. Remove from the heat.

3. Grill the eggplant, fennel, squash, and zucchini on one side until the grill marks are dark brown but the vegetables are still very firm, about 4 minutes. Turn and grill the other side until browned and just tender, about 3 minutes for the squash and zucchini and 5 to 6 minutes longer for the eggplant and fennel. Remove from the heat.

4. Coat the cut sides of the tomatoes with cooking spray. Grill, cut sides down, just until light grill marks appear, about 3 minutes.

5. Heat the oil in a small skillet over medium heat. Add the garlic, marjoram, and remaining ¼ teaspoon salt. Sauté for 1 minute.

6. Peel the grilled pepper and cut it into strips. In a medium bowl, combine the grilled pepper with the rest of the vegetables, then add the olive oil mixture and the vinegar. Toss to coat and serve at room temperature.

PER SERVING **Nutrition info:** 85 calories, 2 g protein, 10 g carbohydrate, 5 g total fat, 1 g saturated fat, 0 mg cholesterol, 4 g fiber, 211 mg sodium

2 Day Diabetes Diet exchanges: 2 vegetable, 1 fat

German Potato Salad with Dijon Vinaigrette

The vinegar in this potato salad helps to slow the absorption of starch into the bloodstream, lowering the glycemic index of this summer treat.

Makes 6 servings

1½ pounds small red potatoes, scrubbed and quartered

½ teaspoon salt, divided

4 slices turkey bacon, cut in half crosswise

1 small onion, chopped

¼ cup apple cider vinegar

2 tablespoons sugar

1 tablespoon coarse-grained Dijon mustard

1 teaspoon olive oil

½ teaspoon freshly ground black pepper

¼ cup finely chopped sweet pickles

¼ cup finely chopped red bell pepper

¼ cup minced parsley

1. Place the potatoes and enough water to cover in a large saucepan. Add ¼ teaspoon of the salt and bring to a boil over high heat. Reduce the heat to medium and cook until tender, about 10 minutes. Drain and keep the potatoes warm.

2. Meanwhile, cook the bacon in a large, deep nonstick skillet until crisp. Drain on paper towels, then crumble. Sauté the onion in the pan juices until golden, about 7 minutes.

3. Shake the vinegar, sugar, mustard, oil, black pepper, and the remaining ¼ teaspoon salt in a jar, then whisk into the skillet. Bring to a simmer and cook until fragrant, about 2 minutes. Add the potatoes, pickles, red pepper, and half of the bacon. Cook, stirring, until the potatoes are evenly coated and heated through, about 2 minutes. Sprinkle with the parsley and the remaining bacon.

PER SERVING **Nutrition info:** 190 calories, 5 g protein, 36 g carbohydrate, 3 g total fat, 1 g saturated fat, 7 mg cholesterol, 3 g fiber, 597 mg sodium

2 Day Diabetes Diet exchanges: ½ vegetable, 2 starch

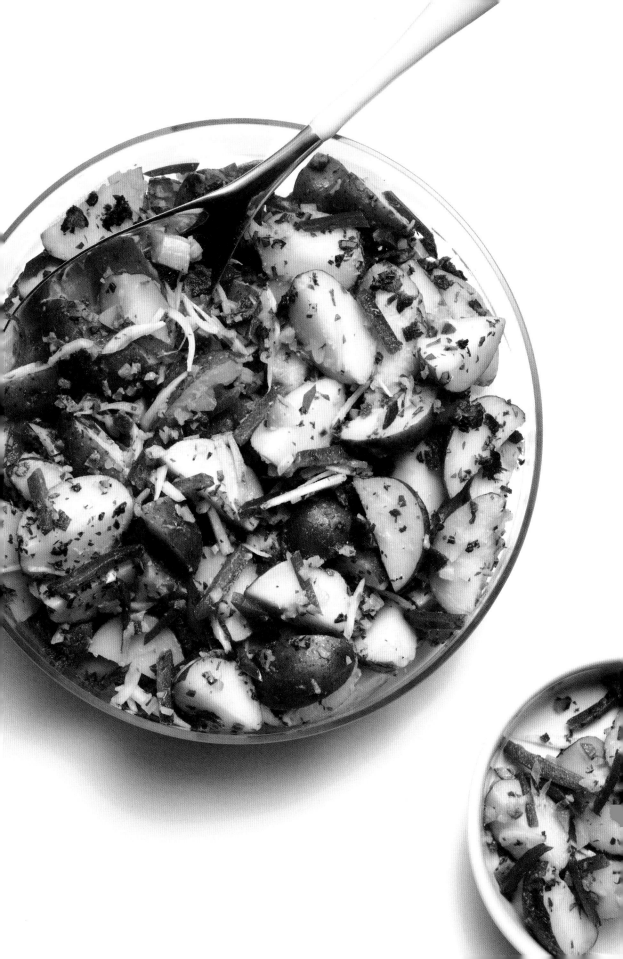

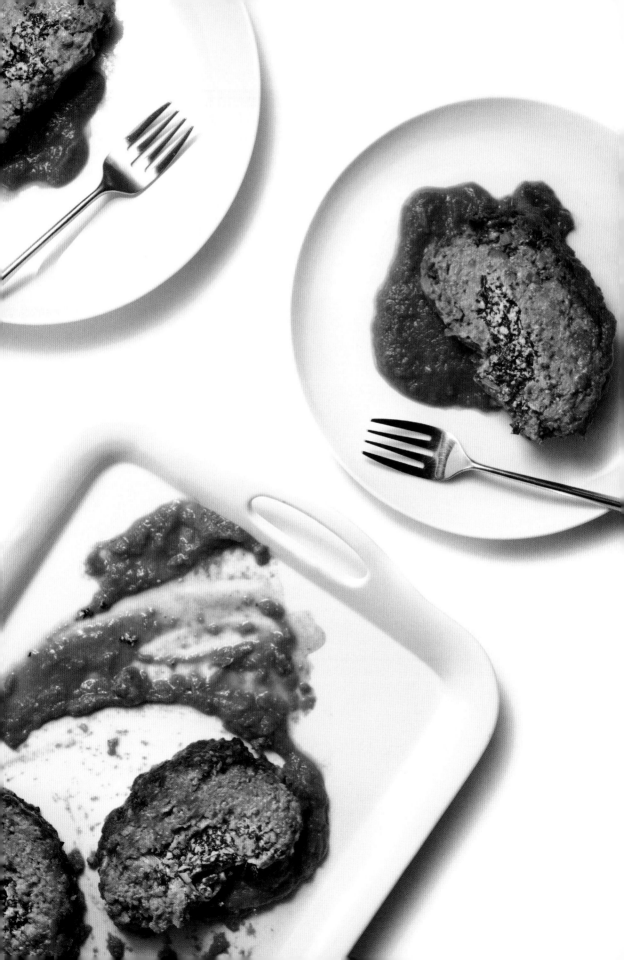

Spinach-Stuffed Meat Loaf

Spinach is not only a great diabetes superfood, it's also a low-calorie extender that can siphon calories out of many fattening dishes, including meat loaf. Along with lean ground turkey, it makes this meat-and-potatoes dish a slimming star.

Makes 6 servings

1 pound lean ground beef

8 ounces lean ground turkey

1 small onion, finely chopped

½ cup fresh bread crumbs

⅛ teaspoon garlic salt

1 tablespoon tomato paste

1 egg white

½ cup part-skim ricotta cheese

1 package (10 ounces) frozen chopped spinach, thawed and drained

⅛ teaspoon salt

⅛ teaspoon ground black pepper

2 large onions, thinly sliced

2 carrots, coarsely chopped

1 can (28 ounces) crushed tomatoes

1. In a bowl, mix the beef, turkey, onion, bread crumbs, garlic salt, and tomato paste. In another bowl, mix the egg white, ricotta, spinach, salt, and pepper.

2. Preheat the oven to 350°F. Turn out the beef mixture onto a large sheet of wax paper, and form it into a 9" x 10" rectangle with your hands.

3. Spoon the spinach stuffing lengthwise down the center of the meat, leaving about 1" of it uncovered at each short end.

4. With the help of the wax paper, lift the long edges of the meat. Fold the meat over the stuffing to enclose it.

5. Using your fingers, pinch the edges of the meat together. Place the loaf seam side down in a nonstick roasting pan. Add the onions, carrots, and tomatoes to the pan.

6. Bake for about 1 ½ hours, or until the meat and vegetables are cooked through. Transfer the meat to a platter. Purée the vegetables in a blender and serve the vegetable sauce with the meat loaf.

PER SERVING **Nutrition info:** 294 calories, 32 g protein, 28 g carbohydrate, 6 g total fat, 2 g saturated fat, 71 mg cholesterol, 2 g fiber, 405 mg sodium

2 Day Diabetes Diet exchanges: 2 vegetable, ½ starch, 5 oz protein

Flank Steak with Red Onions

Flank steak comes from a well-exercised part of the cow, making it naturally lean. Because it's so lean, it's particularly important to marinate this cut of beef before cooking.

Makes 4 servings

- 2 medium red onions, sliced ½" thick
- 2 cloves garlic, crushed
- ⅔ cup balsamic or malt vinegar
- 1 tablespoon olive oil
- 2 tablespoons black currant or seedless raspberry jam
- ½ teaspoon salt
- ½ teaspoon cayenne pepper
- 1 pound flank steak

1. Place the onions, garlic, vinegar, oil, jam, salt, and pepper in a resealable plastic food storage bag. Push out all the air and seal the bag, then knead the marinade through the bag until it is combined. Using a sharp knife and cutting a scant ⅛" deep, score the steak on both sides in a diamond pattern. Add the steak to the marinade, coat the steak well, and reseal the bag. Place the bag on a plate and marinate the steak in the refrigerator for at least 30 minutes or up to 3 hours.

2. Preheat the broiler, setting the rack 5" from the heat. Place an 8" square of aluminum foil on one end of the broiler pan. Using a slotted spoon, remove the onions from the marinade and arrange them on the foil. Place the steak directly on the pan, next to the onions. Broil the onions for 5 minutes on each side, and the steak for 5 to 6 minutes on each side for medium-rare, 7 to 8 minutes for medium. Remove the onions when they are done and keep them warm.

3. Transfer the cooked steak to a cutting board and let stand for 10 minutes, then thinly slice it against the grain, holding the knife at a slight angle. Place the slices on individual plates and spoon any juices over them. Serve with the broiled onions.

PER SERVING **Nutrition info:** 264 calories, 24 g protein, 16 g carbohydrate, 14 g total fat, 6 g saturated fat, 57 mg cholesterol, 1 g fiber, 352 mg sodium

2 Day Diabetes Diet exchanges: ½ vegetable, 1 starch, 4 oz protein, 1 fat

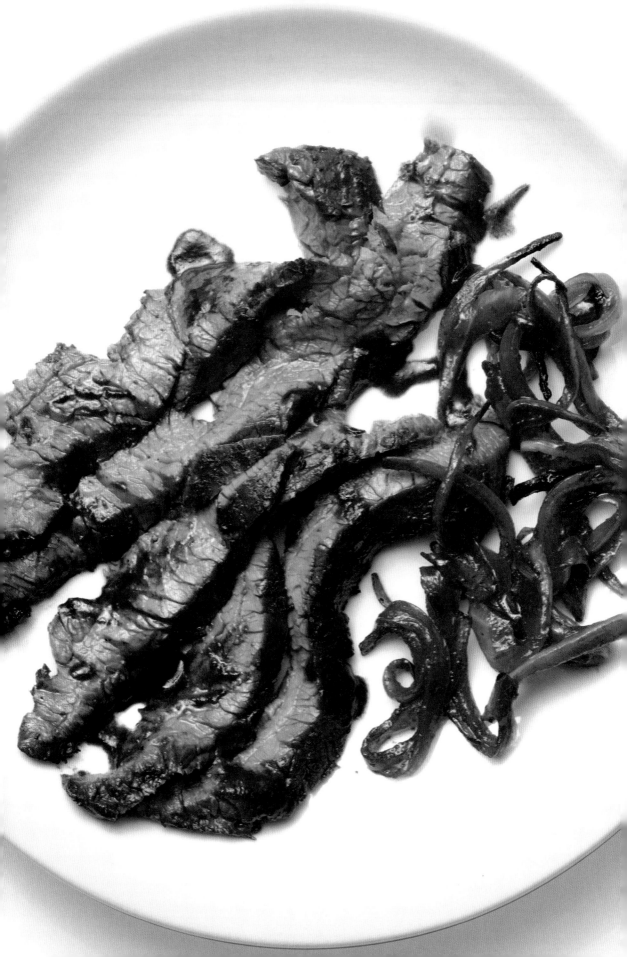

Orange Beef with Broccoli

The varied vegetables in this meal provide a lot of volume for a few calories. Get ready to feast on this Asian-inspired favorite.

Makes 4 servings

- 2 teaspoons cornstarch
- ¼ cup dry sherry
- 2 tablespoons reduced-sodium soy sauce
- ¼ teaspoon baking soda
- 12 ounces flank steak, cut into thin strips
- 4 teaspoons olive oil, divided
- 4 tablespoons finely slivered orange zest, divided
- ¼ teaspoon crushed red-pepper flakes
- 5 cups broccoli florets and stems
- 1 red bell pepper, cut into matchsticks
- 4 scallions, thinly sliced
- 3 cloves garlic, minced
- ½ cup + ⅓ cup water
- 1 cup jicama matchsticks

1. In a medium bowl, whisk together the cornstarch, sherry, soy sauce, and baking soda. Add the steak, tossing to coat. Refrigerate for 30 minutes.

2. In a large nonstick skillet over medium heat, heat 3 teaspoons of the oil. Reserving the marinade, add the beef, 2 tablespoons of the orange zest, and the red-pepper flakes to the skillet. Stir-fry until the beef is just cooked, about 3 minutes. Transfer to a plate.

3. Add the remaining 1 teaspoon oil and the broccoli, bell pepper, scallions, and garlic to the skillet. Cook for 3 minutes longer. Add the ½ cup water. Cook until the broccoli is crisp-tender, about 2 minutes.

4. Stir the ⅓ cup water and reserved marinade into the skillet. Bring to a boil. Cook, stirring, for 1 minute. Return the beef to the skillet. Add the jicama. Cook until the beef is heated through, about 1 minute. Garnish with the remaining 2 tablespoons orange zest.

PER SERVING **Nutrition info:** 284 calories, 21 g protein, 16 g carbohydrate, 14 g total fat, 4 g saturated fat, 16 mg cholesterol, 5 g fiber, 473 mg sodium

2 Day Diabetes Diet exchanges: 2 vegetable, 3 oz protein, 1 fat

Honey-Lime Pork Chops

Pork is a great choice for the budget-conscious cook, as it costs a fraction of the price of other lean meats.

Makes 6 servings (1 chop with 2 tablespoons sauce each)

For the pork chops:

- ½ cup lime juice
- ½ cup reduced-sodium soy sauce
- 2 tablespoons honey
- 2 cloves garlic, minced
- 6 boneless pork loin chops (4 ounces each)

For the sauce:

- ¾ cup reduced-sodium chicken broth
- 1 clove garlic, minced
- 1½ teaspoons honey
- ½ teaspoon lime juice
- ⅛ teaspoon browning sauce

Dash of ground black pepper

- 2 teaspoons cornstarch
- 2 tablespoons water

1. To prepare the pork chops: In a large resealable plastic bag, combine the lime juice, soy sauce, honey, and garlic. Add the pork chops. Seal the bag and turn to coat; refrigerate for 8 hours or overnight.

2. Preheat the grill or broiler. Drain and discard the marinade. Grill the chops, covered, over medium heat or broil 4" from the heat until the juices run clear, 6 to 7 minutes on each side.

3. To prepare the sauce: Combine the broth, garlic, honey, lime juice, browning sauce, and pepper in a small saucepan. Bring to a boil. Combine the cornstarch and water until smooth; stir into the broth mixture. Return to a boil and cook, stirring, for 1 to 2 minutes, or until thickened. Serve with the pork chops.

PER SERVING **Nutrition info:** 200 calories, 26 g protein, 11 g carbohydrate, 5 g total fat, 2 g saturated fat, 71 mg cholesterol, 0 g fiber, 884 mg sodium

2 Day Diabetes Diet exchanges: ½ starch, 4 oz protein

Grilled Chicken Kabobs

This simple summer favorite combines ultra-lean protein with the wholesome bounty of several different types of veggies.

Makes 3 servings (2 skewers per serving)

½ pound boneless, skinless chicken breast, cubed

1 cup chopped bell peppers (1" pieces)

½ cup chopped tomato (1" pieces)

1 cup mushrooms, cut in half

½ cup sliced red onion (1" pieces)

Salt

Ground black pepper

Soak the wooden skewers in water before using. Spray the grill with cooking spray and bring it to medium heat. Thread the chicken, bell peppers, tomato, mushrooms, and onion onto the skewers. Add salt and pepper to taste. Grill for 3 to 4 minutes on each side, or until the chicken is cooked through and reaches an internal temperature of 165°F.

PER SERVING **Nutrition info:** 121 calories, 19 g protein, 8 g carbohydrate, 1 g total fat, 0 g saturated fat, 44 mg cholesterol, 2 g fiber, 293 mg sodium

2 Day Diabetes Diet exchanges: 1 vegetable, 2 oz protein

Curried Chicken Dinner

Curry power is more than a great way to flavor up a dish. Turmeric, one of the spices included in most curry blends, may improve digestion, cool inflammation, ease the pain of arthritis, prevent cancer, and even fend off the germs that make us sick.

Makes 8 servings

8   boneless, skinless chicken breast halves (2 pounds)

½   cup all-purpose flour

2   tablespoons vegetable oil

2   medium onions, chopped

2   medium green bell peppers, chopped

1   clove garlic, minced

2   teaspoons curry powder

½   teaspoon white pepper

2   cans (14 ½ ounces each) diced tomatoes, undrained

1   teaspoon chopped fresh parsley

½   teaspoon dried thyme

1   cup water

3   tablespoons raisins

Hot cooked rice (optional)

1. Preheat the oven to 375°F. Dust the chicken with the flour. In an ovenproof Dutch oven over medium heat, brown the chicken in the oil. Remove the chicken and set aside.

2. Add the onions, bell peppers, and garlic to the drippings and sauté until tender, 3 to 4 minutes. Add the curry and white pepper and mix well. Return the chicken to the Dutch oven. Add the tomatoes, parsley, thyme, and water.

3. Cover and bake for 45 to 50 minutes, or until the chicken is tender and the juices run clear. Stir in the raisins. Serve over rice, if desired.

PER SERVING Nutrition info: 230 calories, 25 g protein, 17 g carbohydrate, 6 g total fat, 1 g saturated fat, 63 mg cholesterol, 2 g fiber, 233 mg sodium

2 Day Diabetes Diet exchanges: 1 vegetable, ½ starch, 3 ½ oz protein, 1 fat

Caribbean Chicken

This recipe contains a perfect blend of hot and sweet. When cutting or seeding hot peppers, use rubber or plastic gloves to protect your hands, and avoid touching your face.

Makes 6 servings

½ cup lemon juice

⅓ cup honey

3 tablespoons canola oil

6 scallions, sliced

3 jalapeño peppers, seeded and chopped

3 teaspoons dried thyme

¾ teaspoon salt

¼ teaspoon ground allspice

¼ teaspoon ground nutmeg

6 boneless, skinless chicken breast halves (1½ pounds)

1. Place the lemon juice, honey, oil, scallions, peppers, thyme, salt, allspice, and nutmeg in a blender or food processor; cover and process until smooth. Pour ½ cup into a small bowl for basting, cover, and refrigerate. Pour the remaining marinade into a large resealable plastic bag and add the chicken. Seal the bag and turn to coat; refrigerate for up to 6 hours.

2. Drain and discard the marinade. Coat a grill rack with cooking spray and preheat the grill. Grill the chicken, covered, over medium heat until the juices run clear, 4 to 6 minutes on each side, basting frequently with the reserved marinade.

PER SERVING Nutrition info: 205 calories, 27 g protein, 11 g carbohydrate, 6 g total fat, 1 g saturated fat, 66 mg cholesterol, 0 g fiber, 272 mg sodium

2 Day Diabetes Diet exchanges: 1 vegetable, ½ starch, 4 oz protein, 1 fat

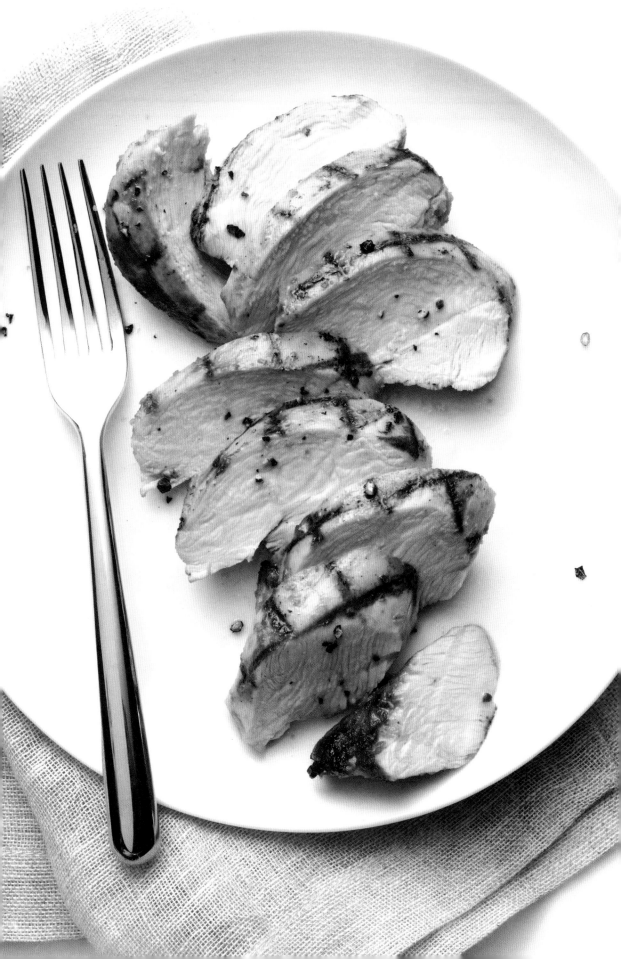

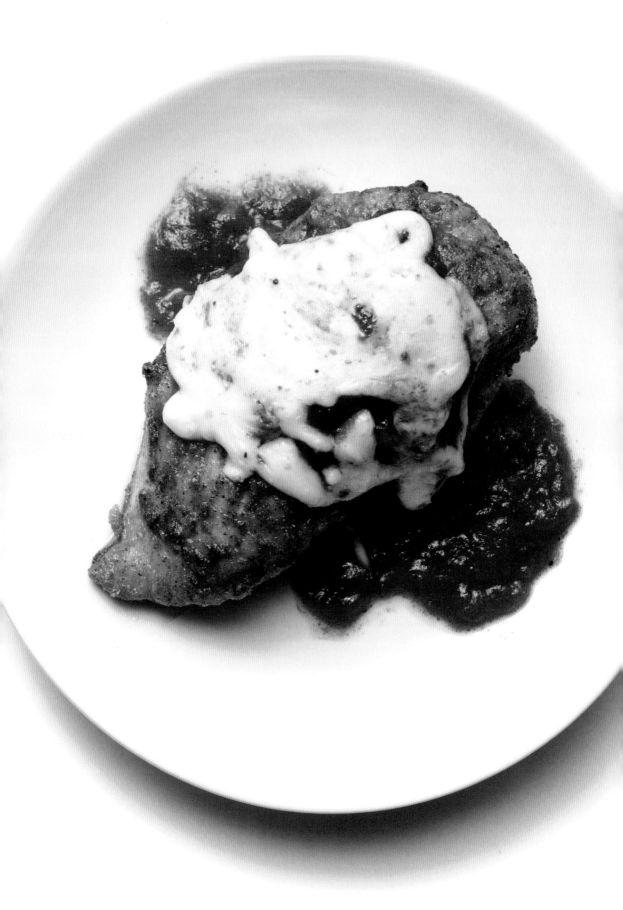

Healthy Chicken Parmesan

Usually Chicken Parmesan is battered and fried—which is precisely the opposite of what you want for optimal health and a slim waistline. This recipe preserves everything you've come to love about this dish while omitting everything that's bad for your health.

Makes 1 serving

- 2 teaspoons olive oil
- 5 ounces boneless, skinless chicken breast
- 3 tablespoons whole-wheat flour
- ¼ cup (1 ounce) shredded fat-free or low-fat mozzarella cheese
- ¼ cup tomato sauce

Place the oil in a sauté pan over medium heat. Dip the chicken breast into the flour and coat both sides evenly. Place the chicken in the pan and cook until both sides are browned and fully cooked through (the internal temperature should reach 165°F). Reduce the heat to low and top the chicken with the tomato sauce and mozzarella. Warm until the cheese melts. Serve warm.

PER SERVING **Nutrition info:** 344 calories, 39 g protein, 23 g carbohydrate, 11 g total fat, 2 g saturated fat, 71 mg cholesterol, 4 g fiber, 788 mg sodium

2 Day Diabetes Diet exchanges: ½ vegetable, 1 starch, 5 oz protein, 2 fat

Grilled Citrus Chicken

This sweet, mustardy marinade turns same old, same old chicken into an extraordinary summer delight.

Makes 6 servings

6   boneless, skinless chicken breast halves (1 ½ pounds)

½   cup packed brown sugar

¼   cup apple cider vinegar

3   tablespoons lemon juice

3   tablespoons lime juice

3   tablespoons Dijon mustard

¾   teaspoon garlic powder

¼   teaspoon ground black pepper

1. Place the chicken in a shallow glass dish. Combine the sugar, vinegar, lemon juice, lime juice, mustard, garlic powder, and pepper and pour the mixture over the chicken. Cover and refrigerate for 4 hours or overnight.

2. Preheat the grill. Drain the chicken, discarding the marinade. Grill the chicken over medium-hot coals, turning once, until the juices run clear, about 15 to 18 minutes.

PER SERVING **Nutrition info:** 200 calories, 26 g protein, 20 g carbohydrate, 2 g total fat, 1 g saturated fat, 20 mg cholesterol, 0 g fiber, 180 mg sodium

2 Day Diabetes Diet exchanges: 1 starch, 4 oz protein

Salmon on a Bed of Greens

The combination of omega-3-rich salmon and nutrient-loaded kale makes this dish a standout when it comes to total body health.

Makes 4 servings

¼ cup grapefruit juice

1½ tablespoons mustard

1½ tablespoons honey

¼ teaspoon red-pepper flakes

4 salmon fillets (6 ounces each)

2 quarts water

1½ pounds kale, large stems removed and leaves chopped

3 tablespoons olive oil

½ red bell pepper, seeded and finely chopped

½ yellow pepper, seeded and finely chopped

1. In a baking dish large enough to hold fish fillets in a single layer, combine the grapefruit juice, mustard, honey, and red-pepper flakes. Add the salmon to the dish, turning to coat both sides with the marinade. Refrigerate, covered, for 30 minutes.

2. Preheat the broiler.

3. In a large pot, bring the water to a boil. Add the kale. Return the water to a boil and cook for 5 minutes. Drain well. Squeeze out any excess water.

4. Heat the oil in a large skillet over medium heat. Add the red and yellow bell peppers and sauté for 1 minute. Add the kale. Sauté until the peppers and kale are tender, about 3 minutes. Remove the skillet from the heat and keep warm.

5. Remove the salmon from the marinade. Place, skin side down, on a rack in a foil-lined broiler pan. Reserve the marinade.

6. Broil the salmon 4" from the heat for 3 minutes. Brush on the remaining marinade. Broil until the fish is opaque and flakes when touched with a knife, 3 to 4 minutes. Serve the salmon on a bed of the kale and peppers.

PER SERVING **Nutrition info:** 402 calories, 41 g protein, 21 g carbohydrate, 18 g total fat, 3 g saturated fat, 97 mg cholesterol, 3 g fiber, 233 mg sodium

2 Day Diabetes Diet exchanges: 1 vegetable, ½ starch, 6 oz protein, 2 fat

Sunshine Halibut

This firm, meaty fish tastes sweet—a flavor that this recipe accentuates with orange juice and zest. Like salmon and other cold-water fish, halibut is a rich source of healthy omega-3 fatty acids.

Makes 4 servings

⅓ cup chopped onion

1 clove garlic, minced

2 tablespoons minced fresh parsley

½ teaspoon grated orange zest

4 halibut steaks (4 ounces each)

¼ cup orange juice

1 tablespoon lemon juice

¼ teaspoon salt

¼ teaspoon lemon-pepper seasoning

1. Preheat the oven to 400°F. In a nonstick skillet coated with cooking spray, sauté the onion and garlic until tender; remove from the heat. Stir in the parsley and orange zest.

2. Place the halibut in an 8" square baking dish coated with cooking spray. Top with the onion mixture.

3. Combine the orange and lemon juices and pour over the fish. Sprinkle with the salt and lemon-pepper seasoning. Cover and bake until the fish flakes easily with a fork, 15 to 20 minutes.

PER SERVING Nutrition info: 142 calories, 24 g protein, 4 g carbohydrate, 3 g total fat, 0 g saturated fat, 36 mg cholesterol, 0 g fiber, 237 mg sodium

2 Day Diabetes Diet exchanges: 4 oz protein

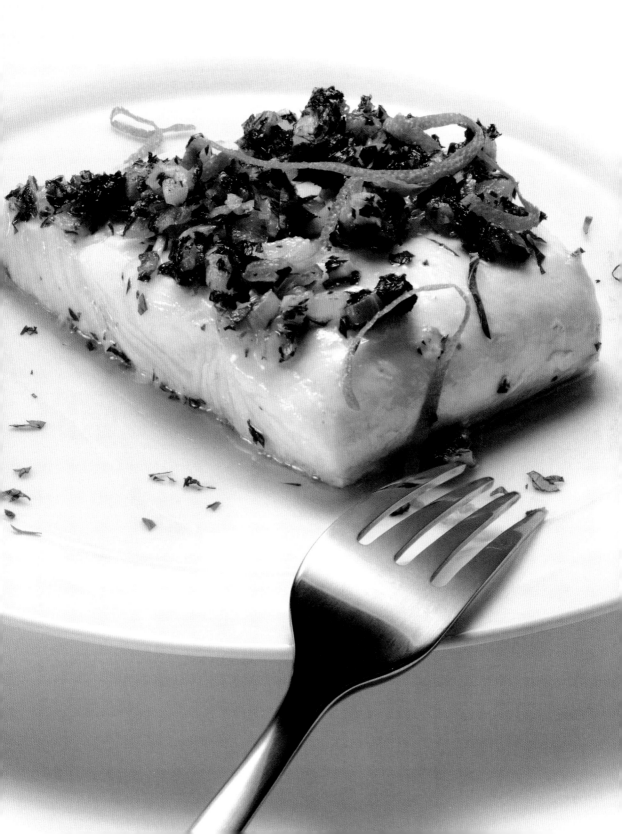

Baked Cod Casserole with Potatoes, Tomatoes, and Arugula

This combination of lean cod with nutrient-dense veggies allows you to consume a huge portion of food for only a minimal number of calories.

Makes 4 servings

1	pound red potatoes, unpeeled and cut into ½"-thick slices
1	onion, thinly sliced
1	tablespoon olive oil
½	teaspoon salt, divided
4	plum tomatoes, seeded and coarsely chopped
3	cloves garlic, minced
½	teaspoon dried oregano, crumbled
1½	cups arugula
1	pound cod, scrod, halibut, or other thick, firm-fleshed white fish steaks, cut into 2" chunks

1. 1. Preheat the oven to 350°F. In a 13" x 9" baking dish, combine the potatoes, onion, oil, and ¼ teaspoon of the salt.

2. Bake for 20 minutes, stirring the mixture once.

3. Stir the tomatoes, garlic, and oregano into the potato mixture. Spread the arugula on top in an even layer. Top with the cod. Sprinkle with the remaining ¼ teaspoon salt.

4. Bake, covered with aluminum foil, just until the fish is cooked through, 15 to 18 minutes. Transfer the fish and vegetable mixture to serving plates. Spoon the pan juices over each serving.

PER SERVING Nutrition info: 213 calories, 22 g protein, 21 g carbohydrate, 5 g total fat, 1 g saturated fat, 43 mg cholesterol, 4 g fiber, 363 mg sodium

2 Day Diabetes Diet exchanges: 1 vegetable, 1 starch, 3 oz protein, 1 fat

Walnut-Encrusted Tilapia

One of the most common types of farmed fish, tilapia is flaky, light and the perfect fish to consume if you are on a tight budget. The walnuts add some healthy omega-3 fatty acids to what is otherwise an ultra-lean recipe.

Makes 1 serving

3 tablespoons whole-wheat flour

1 tablespoon crushed walnuts

1 tilapia fillet (5 ounces)

1 tablespoon olive oil

1. In a medium bowl, mix together the flour and walnuts.

2. Dip the tilapia into the flour mixture and coat both sides evenly.

3. Add the oil to a sauté pan and place it over medium heat.

4. Place the coated tilapia in the pan and cook both sides evenly until cooked through (the tilapia should have an opaque color throughout). Serve warm.

PER SERVING **Nutrition info:** 300 calories, 33 g protein, 18 g carbohydrate, 12 g total fat, 2 g saturated fat, 71 mg cholesterol, 3 g fiber, 76 mg sodium

2 Day Diabetes Diet exchanges: 1 starch, 5 oz protein, 2 fat

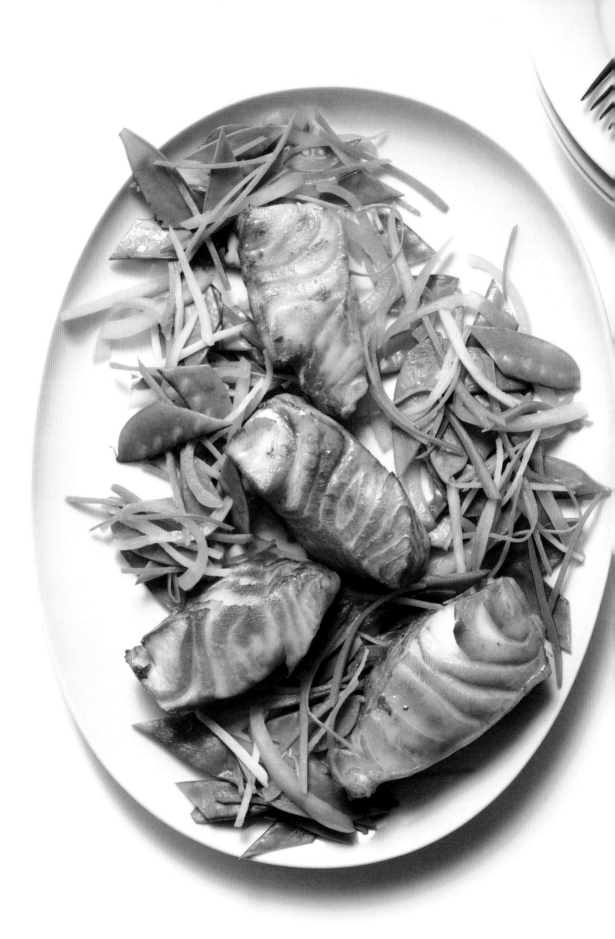

Asian Steamed Fish Fillets with Vegetable Sticks

The snow peas in this recipe don't just taste fantastic. They contain a nutrient called coumestrol, which is thought to reduce risk for stomach cancer. Other nutrients in these important vegetables offer anti-inflammatory benefits.

Makes 4 servings

- 4 halibut or other firm-fleshed white fish fillets (1½ pounds total)
- 2 tablespoons soy sauce
- 2 tablespoons white wine or sake
- 1 thin slice peeled fresh ginger, cut into thin matchsticks
- 2 medium carrots, cut into 3" x ¼" matchsticks
- 2 ounces snow peas, cut in half lengthwise
- ½ yellow bell pepper, seeded and cut into thin matchsticks

1. Place the fillets in a baking dish that will fit inside a large steamer basket or on a rack that will fit into a large skillet. In a small cup, stir together the soy sauce and wine. Pour over the fish. Top with the ginger and carrots.

2. Fill the skillet with 1" of water. Bring to a simmer. Place the steamer basket or wire rack in the skillet.

3. Place the baking dish containing the fish in the steamer basket or on the wire rack. Cover. Steam for 5 to 6 minutes.

4. Add the snow peas and yellow pepper to the baking dish and again cover it. Steam until the fish flakes when touched with a fork and the vegetables are crisp-tender, about 5 minutes. Serve at once.

PER SERVING **Nutrition info:** 175 calories, 32 g protein, 7 g carbohydrate, 3 g total fat, 0 g saturated fat, 45 mg cholesterol, 2 g fiber, 558 mg sodium

2 Day Diabetes Diet exchanges: 1 vegetable, 5 oz protein

Zippy Shrimp

Paprika, one of the spices in this recipe, contains important carotenoids. Other than turning the entire dish a vibrant shade of orange, this nutrient fights inflammation, as do the array of nutrients found in red chiles. When cutting or seeding the chiles, use rubber or plastic gloves to protect your hands. Avoid touching your face.

Makes 8 servings (½ cup each)

1¼ cups chicken or vegetable broth

10 medium pitted ripe olives, finely chopped

1 red chile pepper, finely chopped

2 tablespoons lemon juice

1 tablespoon minced fresh rosemary or 1 teaspoon dried rosemary, crushed

4 cloves garlic, minced

2 teaspoons Worcestershire sauce

1 teaspoon paprika

½ teaspoon salt

¼–½ teaspoon ground black pepper

2 pounds fresh or frozen uncooked shrimp, peeled and deveined

1. In a large nonstick skillet, combine the broth, olives, chile pepper, lemon juice, rosemary, garlic, Worcestershire sauce, paprika, salt, and black pepper. Bring to a boil and cook until the mixture is reduced by half.

2. Add the shrimp. Simmer, uncovered, for 3 to 4 minutes or until the shrimp turn pink, stirring occasionally.

PER SERVING **Nutrition info:** 141 calories, 24 g protein, 3 g carbohydrate, 3 g total fat, 0 g saturated fat, 172 mg cholesterol, 0 g fiber, 520 mg sodium

2 Day Diabetes Diet exchanges: 3 ½ oz protein

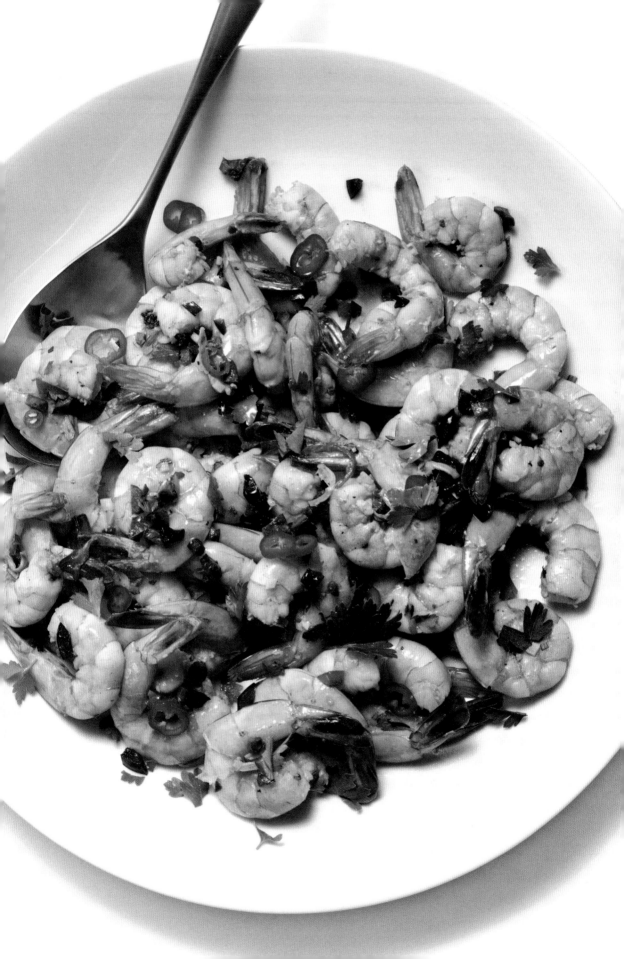

Bean and Vegetable Tostadas

Mexican food wouldn't be Mexican without some heat. Just be careful when cutting and seeding the jalapeño pepper. Use rubber or plastic gloves to protect your hands. Avoid touching your face.

Makes 6 servings (1 tostada each)

6   corn tortillas (6" diameter)

1   can (15 ounces) black beans, drained and rinsed

1   can (11 ounces) corn kernels, drained and rinsed

1   small tomato, cored and chopped (about ½ cup)

2   tablespoons finely chopped red onion

1   small jalapeño pepper, seeded and finely chopped

2   tablespoons chopped cilantro

1   tablespoon freshly squeezed lime juice

½   teaspoon salt

⅛-¼ teaspoon hot red-pepper sauce

1   small ripe avocado, pitted, peeled, and chopped

1. Preheat the oven to 450°F. Place the tortillas in a single layer on 2 baking sheets. Coat both sides of tortillas with cooking spray. Bake until lightly browned and crisp, about 10 minutes, flipping the tortillas over halfway through. Transfer to wire racks and let cool.

2. In a large bowl, stir together the beans, corn, tomato, onion, jalapeño, cilantro, lime juice, salt, and hot sauce. Gently fold in the avocado. Spoon ½ cup of the mixture onto each tortilla.

PER SERVING Nutrition info: 130 calories, 5 g protein, 26 g carbohydrate, 1 g total fat, 0 g saturated fat, 0 mg cholesterol, 5 g fiber, 390 mg sodium

2 Day Diabetes Diet exchanges: ½ vegetable, 1 ½ starch, 1 oz protein

Portabella Mushroom Pizza

Portabella mushrooms are the "meats" of the vegetable kingdom. They add a meaty texture to this great vegetarian option.

Makes 1 serving

1　large portabella mushroom

½　cup (2 ounces) fat-free or low-fat mozzarella cheese

2　tablespoons no-salt-added tomato paste

½　cup diced tomatoes

1　teaspoon dried oregano

¼　teaspoon garlic powder

Preheat the grill. Grill the portabella mushroom over medium heat until tender. Top the mushroom with the cheese, tomato paste, tomatoes, oregano, and garlic powder. Heat on the grill (or in a microwave oven) until the cheese is melted. Serve warm.

PER SERVING **Nutrition info:** 158 calories, 22 g protein, 19 g carbohydrate, 1 g total fat, 0 g saturated fat, 10 mg cholesterol, 4 g fiber, 726 mg sodium

2 Day Diabetes Diet exchanges: 2 vegetable, 2 oz protein

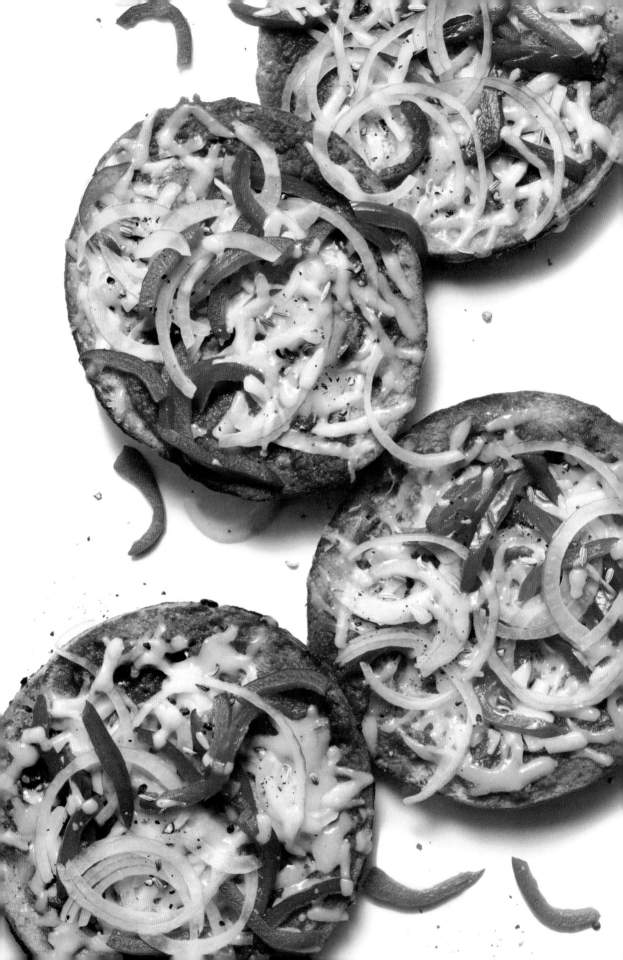

Pita Pizza

Regular pizza dough is loaded with carbs and calories, but this version uses naturally low-carb and low-calorie pita. The end result: satisfaction without the blood-sugar-raising carbs.

Makes 4 servings

½ cup thinly sliced roasted red bell peppers

¼ teaspoon crushed fennel seeds or dried oregano, crumbled

¼ teaspoon salt

⅛ teaspoon ground black pepper

¼ cup (1 ounce) shredded reduced-fat mozzarella cheese

2 tablespoons (½ ounce) shredded Gruyère or Jarlsberg cheese

2 whole-wheat pitas (4" diameter)

8 teaspoons bottled tomato sauce or pizza sauce

½ small red onion, thinly sliced

1. Preheat the broiler.

2. In a small bowl, combine the red peppers, fennel or oregano, salt, and pepper. In a second bowl, combine the mozzarella and Gruyère or Jarlsberg.

3. Separate each pita into 2 flat rounds. Place the rounds, rough side up, on a baking sheet. Broil 4" from the heat until golden brown around the edges, about 1 minute. Remove from the broiler.

4. Spread 2 teaspoons sauce over each pita, covering to the edges. Spoon 2 tablespoons red pepper mixture over each pita. Sprinkle with cheese, dividing equally among the pitas, then add the onion in rings.

5. Broil until the cheese is melted and the pizzas are hot, about 2 minutes.

PER SERVING **Nutrition info:** 137 calories, 7 g protein, 23 g carbohydrate, 3 g total fat, 2 g saturated fat, 7 mg cholesterol, 3 g fiber, 475 mg sodium

2 Day Diabetes Diet exchanges: ½ vegetable, ½ starch, ½ oz protein

Eggplant Lasagna

Normally lasagna is brimming with gooey, fattening cheese. This version uses lean silken tofu to maintain the wonderful gooey texture but slash the fat and calories.

Makes 12 servings

2   tablespoons olive oil

1   large onion, chopped

2   cloves garlic, minced

1   tablespoon Italian seasoning

2   cans (14 ounces each) diced tomatoes

1   can (28 ounces) tomato sauce

1   small eggplant, peeled and cut into 1" pieces

¼   teaspoon salt

1   container (16 ounces) light silken tofu, drained

2   large eggs

1   cup (4 ounces) grated Parmesan cheese

9   no-boil lasagna noodles

2   cups (8 ounces) shredded part-skim mozzarella cheese

1. Preheat the oven to 400°F. Heat the oil in a large saucepan over medium-high heat. Add the onion and cook until tender, about 5 minutes. Add the garlic and Italian seasoning and cook for 1 minute longer. Add the tomatoes and tomato sauce and bring to a simmer. Reduce the heat to low and simmer until the flavors are blended, about 40 minutes.

2. Meanwhile, coat a baking sheet with cooking spray. Add the eggplant, coat it with cooking spray, and sprinkle it with the salt. Roast, turning occasionally, for 30 minutes, or until browned.

3. In a food processor, combine the tofu, eggs, and Parmesan and puree until smooth.

4. Coat a 13" x 9" baking dish with cooking spray. Spread 1 cup sauce in the dish and arrange 3 lasagna noodles on top. Spread half of the tofu filling over the noodles, followed by half of the eggplant. Top with 1 ½ cups sauce and ½ cup mozzarella. Repeat with another layer, then top with the remaining noodles, sauce, and mozzarella.

5. Cover with foil and bake for 1 hour. Remove the foil and bake until heated through, about 15 minutes. Let cool slightly before serving.

PER SERVING **Nutrition info:** 229 calories, 16 g protein, 10 g total fat, 4 g saturated fat, 51 mg cholesterol, 3 g fiber, 19 g carbohydrates, 852 mg sodium

2 Day Diabetes Diet exchanges: 1 ½ vegetable, ¼ starch, 1 ½ oz protein, 2 fat

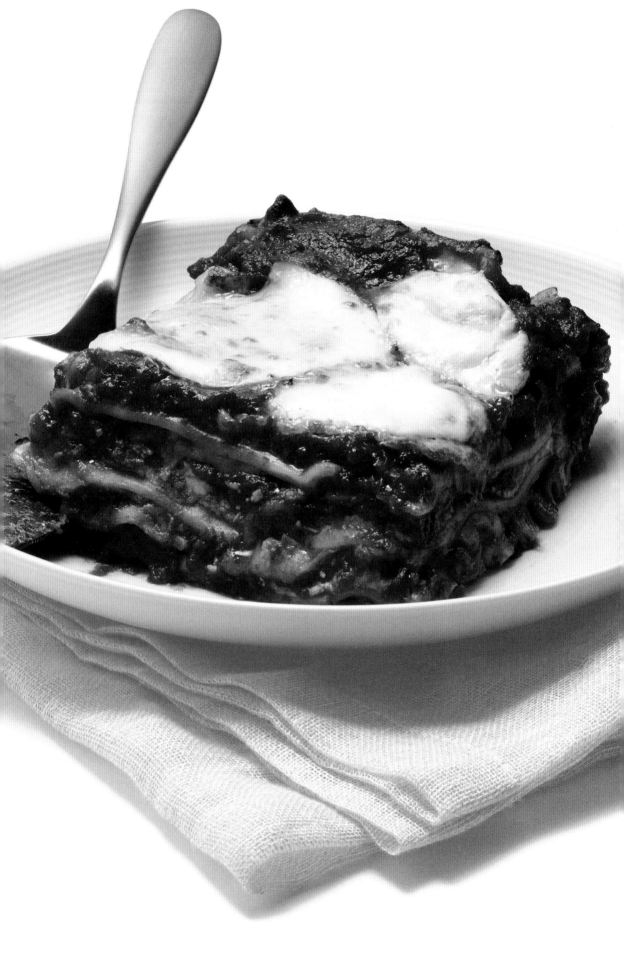

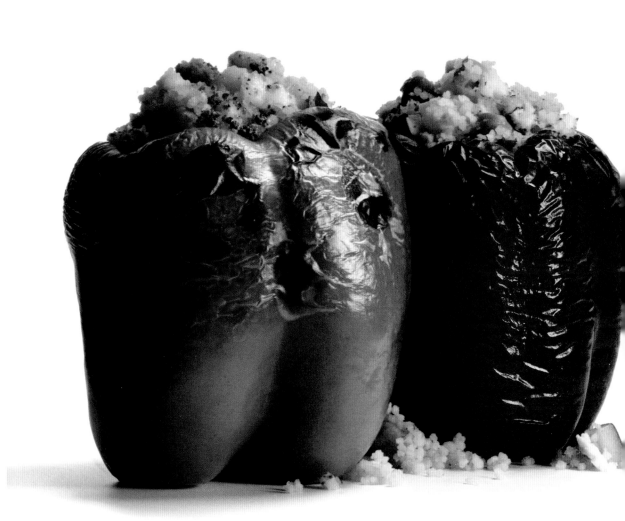

Couscous-Stuffed Peppers

Garbanzo beans are loaded with appetite-suppressing fiber, which is why this dish satisfies your appetite on so few calories.

Makes 6 servings

6   large bell peppers (red, yellow, orange, or green)

1   tablespoon vegetable oil

1   small zucchini, finely chopped

2   cloves garlic, minced

1   tablespoon freshly squeezed lemon juice

2   cups cooked couscous

1   can (15 ounces) garbanzo beans, drained and rinsed

1   ripe tomato, seeded and finely chopped

1   teaspoon dried oregano, crumbled

½   teaspoon salt

¼   teaspoon ground black pepper

½   cup crumbled feta cheese

1. Slice the tops off the peppers to make lids. Scoop out the membranes and seeds and discard. In a large saucepan of lightly salted boiling water, simmer the peppers and lids, covered, for 5 minutes. Drain.

2. Preheat the oven to 350°F.

3. Heat the oil in a medium saucepan over medium heat. Add the zucchini and garlic. Sauté for 2 minutes. Stir in the lemon juice. Cook for 1 minute and remove from heat. Stir in the couscous, garbanzo beans, tomato, oregano, salt, and pepper. Stir in the cheese. Fill each pepper with the couscous mixture. Place the peppers upright in a shallow baking dish. Cover with the pepper tops.

4. Bake just until the filling is heated through, about 20 minutes.

PER SERVING **Nutrition info:** 207 calories, 8 g protein, 36 g carbohydrate, 4 g total fat, 1 g saturated fat, 3 mg cholesterol, 7 g fiber, 307 mg sodium

2 Day Diabetes Diet exchanges: 1 ½ vegetable, 2 starch, 1 oz protein, ½ fat

Barley Risotto with Asparagus and Mushrooms

Usually risotto is made from high-starch white rice, but this recipe uses fiber-rich barley and pairs it with low-starch veggies to create a delicious blood-sugar-friendly dish.

Makes 4 servings

2 cans (14 ½ ounces each) reduced-sodium, fat-free chicken broth

2 cups water

2 tablespoons olive oil

1 onion, finely chopped

8 ounces mushrooms, preferably a mixture of wild varieties, coarsely chopped

2 cloves garlic, minced

1 cup pearl barley

8 ounces asparagus, trimmed and cut into bite-size pieces, leaving tips whole

½ cup (2 ounces) grated Parmesan cheese

1. In a medium saucepan, heat the broth and water to just below a simmer. Cover and keep at a simmer.

2. In a large, deep nonstick skillet over medium heat, heat the oil. Sauté the onion until slightly softened, about 3 minutes. Add the mushrooms and garlic. Sauté until the mushrooms are softened, about 5 minutes. Stir in the barley and then 2 cups of the hot broth mixture. Simmer, covered, for 15 minutes.

3. Meanwhile, blanch the asparagus tips in the pot of hot broth for 2 minutes. Transfer with a slotted spoon to a plate.

4. Add more hot broth to the barley mixture, ½ cup at a time, stirring frequently. Let each batch of liquid be absorbed before adding more. When adding the last batch of liquid, stir in the asparagus stem pieces. Stir in the Parmesan. Serve the risotto topped with the asparagus tips.

PER SERVING **Nutrition info:** 329 calories, 15 g protein, 49 g carbohydrate, 10 g total fat, 2 g saturated fat, 23 mg cholesterol, 10 g fiber, 743 mg sodium

2 Day Diabetes Diet exchanges: 2 vegetable, 1 starch, 2 oz protein, 2 fat

Penne with Fresh Tomato Sauce and Grilled Eggplant

They don't garner as much news play as many other types of produce, but that doesn't mean that eggplants are not incredibly good for you. They are rich in chlorogenic acid, a nutrient thought to prevent both heart disease and cancer.

Makes 4 servings

- 1 eggplant (1 pound), cut lengthwise into ¾"-thick slices
- ½ teaspoon salt, divided
- 2 tablespoons olive oil
- 4 cloves garlic, thinly sliced
- 1½ pounds ripe plum tomatoes, halved, seeded, and coarsely chopped
- 1 teaspoon chopped fresh oregano or ½ teaspoon dried, crumbled
- 2 teaspoons balsamic vinegar
- ½ teaspoon sugar
- 8 ounces penne pasta
- ¼ cup (1 ounce) shaved or shredded Parmesan cheese

1. Sprinkle the eggplant with ¼ teaspoon of the salt. Let stand for at least 30 minutes to draw out liquid.

2. Meanwhile, heat the oil in a large nonstick skillet over medium-low heat. Add the garlic and cook, stirring, for 1 minute. Add the tomatoes, oregano, and the remaining ¼ teaspoon of salt. Increase the heat to medium and cook just until the tomatoes are softened, about 6 minutes. Stir in the vinegar and sugar and cook for 30 seconds longer.

3. Preheat the grill or broiler. Rinse the eggplant and pat dry. Lightly spray both sides of the slices with cooking spray. Grill or broil 4" from the heat until softened and, if grilling, dark grill marks appear, about 5 minutes on each side. Set aside to cool slightly.

4. Meanwhile, cook the pasta according to package directions. Drain and toss with the tomato mixture. Coarsely chop the eggplant and add it to the pasta, then stir in the cheese. Serve hot or at room temperature.

PER SERVING **Nutrition info:** 360 calories, 13 g protein, 59 g carbohydrate, 10 g total fat, 2 g saturated fat, 4 mg cholesterol, 7 g fiber, 406 mg sodium

2 Day Diabetes Diet exchanges: 1 starch, 1 oz protein

Rigatoni with Broccoli Rabe, Cherry Tomatoes, and Roasted Garlic

A staple in Italian cooking, broccoli rabe is one of the world's richest sources of glucosinolates, important nutrients that are known to fend off cancer.

Makes 4 servings

12 ounces rigatoni

2 small bunches broccoli rabe, tough stems removed and leaves cut crosswise into 1"-wide pieces

1 tablespoon olive oil

1 red onion, halved and thinly sliced crosswise

1 yellow bell pepper, seeded and cut lengthwise into thin strips

2 scallions, thinly sliced on the diagonal

½ cup golden raisins

¼ teaspoon red-pepper flakes

¼ teaspoon salt

8 cloves roasted garlic

12 cherry tomatoes, halved

Pinch of ground nutmeg

¼ teaspoon freshly ground black pepper

¼ cup (1 ounce) grated Parmesan cheese

1. Cook the rigatoni according to package directions. Add the broccoli rabe to the pot for the last 5 minutes of cooking. Drain and remove from pot.

2. Meanwhile, heat the oil in a large nonstick skillet over medium-high heat. Add the onion, bell pepper, scallions, raisins, pepper flakes, and salt. Sauté until crisp-tender, about 4 minutes. Add the garlic and sauté for 1 minute longer. Remove from the heat.

3. Return the pasta and broccoli rabe to the pot. Stir in the pepper mixture, tomatoes, and nutmeg. Sprinkle with the black pepper and cheese.

PER SERVING **Nutrition info:** 515 calories, 21 g protein, 98 g carbohydrate, 7 g total fat, 2 g saturated fat, 4 mg cholesterol, 6 g fiber, 506 mg sodium

2 Day Diabetes Diet exchanges: 1 ½ vegetable, 1 fruit, 3 starch, 2 oz protein, 1 fat

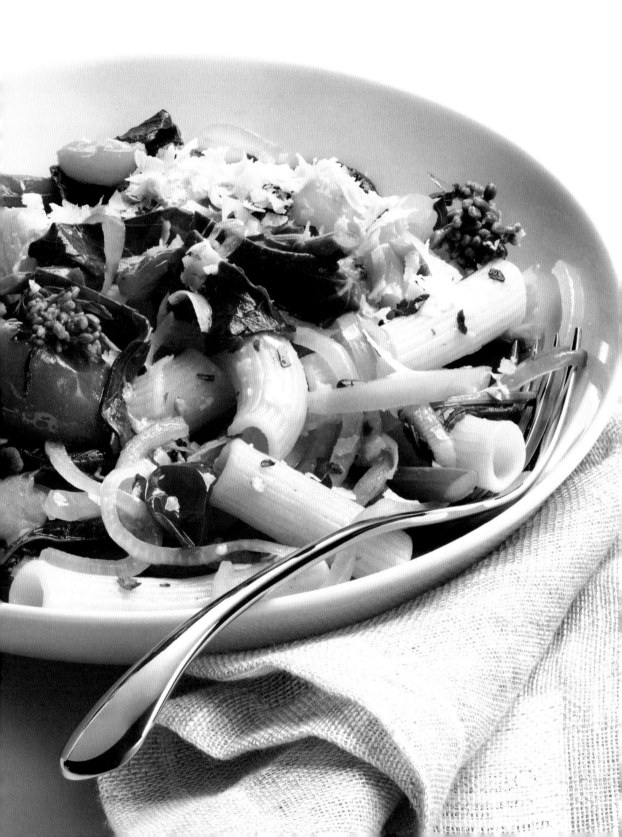

Cold Sesame Noodles and Vegetables

This satisfying pasta salad offers an exotic Asian accent. It's loaded with fiber-rich vegetables that will fill you up on very few calories.

Makes 6 servings

8 ounces whole-wheat linguine

⅓ cup cilantro leaves

2 tablespoons peanut butter

2 tablespoons reduced-sodium soy sauce

2½ teaspoons honey

1 tablespoon rice vinegar or apple cider vinegar

1 tablespoon dark sesame oil

2 cloves garlic, peeled

½ teaspoon salt

¼ teaspoon cayenne pepper

2 carrots, slivered

1 red bell pepper, slivered

1 large stalk celery, slivered

2 scallions, slivered

1. Cook the linguine in a large pot of boiling water according to package directions. Drain, reserving ½ cup of the cooking water.

2. Combine the cilantro, peanut butter, soy sauce, honey, vinegar, sesame oil, garlic, salt, and cayenne in a food processor. Puree. Transfer to a large bowl.

3. Whisk in the reserved pasta-cooking water. Add the linguine, carrots, bell pepper, celery, and scallions. Toss. Chill at least 1 hour before serving.

PER SERVING **Nutrition info:** 200 calories, 7 g protein, 33 g carbohydrate, 5.5 g total fat, 1 g saturated fat, 0 mg cholesterol, 6 g fiber, 422 mg sodium

2 Day Diabetes Diet exchanges: 1 vegetable, 1 ½ starch, 1 fat

Steamed Sesame Spinach

One of the superfoods on the 2 Day Diabetes Diet, spinach is a great green to always have on hand. Steam it in a bag or try it in this simple side dish.

Makes 4 servings

1 pound spinach, stems removed

⅛ teaspoon red-pepper flakes

½ teaspoon dark sesame oil

1 teaspoon salt

1 teaspoon freshly squeezed lemon juice

1 tablespoon sesame seeds, toasted

1. In a medium saucepan, steam the spinach with the pepper flakes until tender, 3 to 5 minutes. Transfer to a serving bowl.

2. Add the sesame oil, salt, and lemon juice to the spinach. Toss to mix. Sprinkle with the sesame seeds. Serve at once.

PER SERVING **Nutrition info:** 38 calories, 3 g protein, 4 g carbohydrate, 2 g total fat, 0 g saturated fat, 0 mg cholesterol, 3 g fiber, 43 mg sodium

2 Day Diabetes Diet exchanges: 1 vegetable

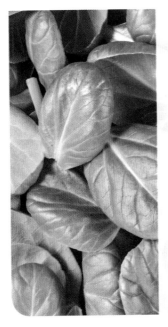

SUPERFOOD SPOTLIGHT: Spinach

Spinach is one of many leafy greens (collards are another great choice) that have been shown to drop the risk of developing diabetes. People who consume more than 1 serving a day of spinach and other leafy greens slashed their risk by 14 percent compared to people who ate less than ½ serving daily, found one British study.[3] This green is particularly rich in vitamin K, along with several minerals: magnesium, folate, phosphorus, potassium, and zinc. It's also a good source of the plant chemicals lutein and zeaxanthin and various flavonoids. Although spinach is technically a rich source of calcium, another nutrient in spinach called oxalic acid prevents much of that calcium from being absorbed unless you use this quick tip: Blanch spinach by boiling it for just 1 minute to reduce this chemical. Spinach is one of those versatile vegetables that you can throw into anything: soups, salads, omelets, smoothies, wraps. Keep a bag of prewashed spinach on hand, and toss it in at the last minute.

Roasted Asparagus and Red Pepper with Parmesan

This is a great spring recipe, perfect for when these delectable asparagus shoots are emerging from the ground. Loaded with fiber, folate, and vitamins, asparagus is a standout source of chromium, a trace mineral that helps insulin more easily transport sugar into cells.

Makes 4 servings

- 1 pound asparagus, trimmed and bottom halves of stalks thinly peeled
- 1 red bell pepper, seeded and cut lengthwise into thin strips
- 1 tablespoon olive oil
- 1 tablespoon balsamic vinegar
- 1 piece (1 ounce) Parmesan cheese
- ¼ teaspoon ground black pepper

1. Preheat the oven to 500°F.

2. Place the asparagus and bell pepper strips in large shallow baking pan. Drizzle with oil. Toss to coat.

3. Roast until crisp-tender, 10 to 12 minutes, turning occasionally. Transfer to a serving dish.

4. Sprinkle with vinegar. Toss to coat. Using a vegetable peeler, shave the cheese into thin curls over the vegetables. Season with the black pepper.

PER SERVING **Nutrition info:** 86 calories, 5 g protein, 5 g carbohydrate, 6 g total fat, 2 g saturated fat, 6 mg cholesterol, 2 g fiber, 140 mg sodium

2 Day Diabetes Diet exchanges: 1 vegetable, 1 fat

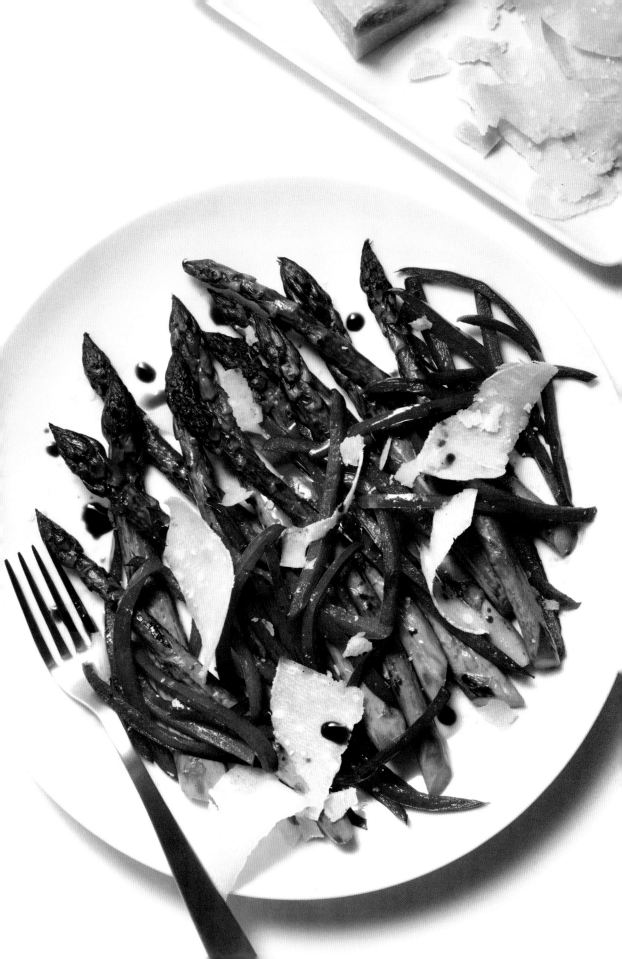

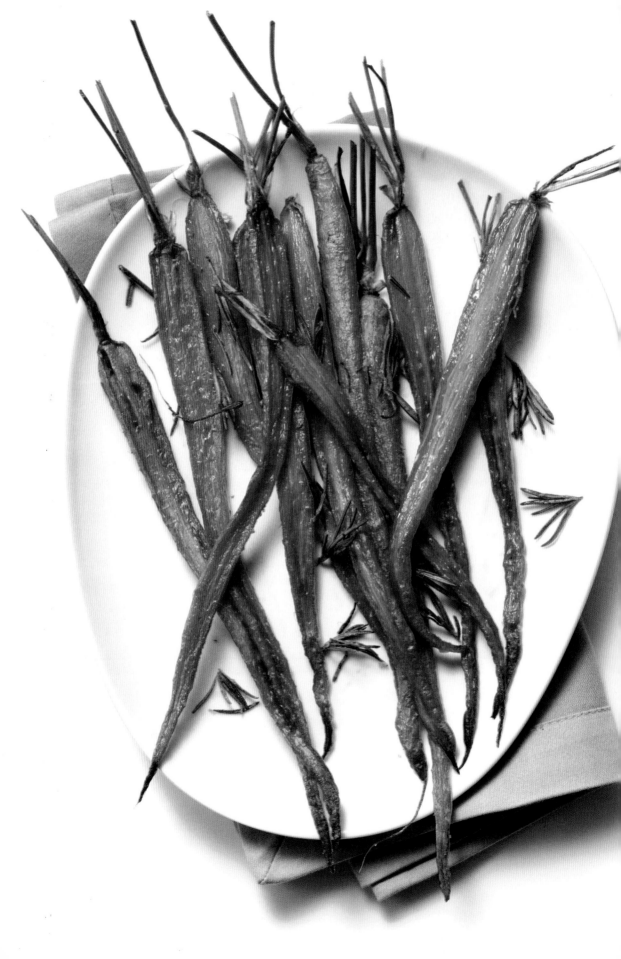

Roasted Carrots with Rosemary

Orange vegetables like carrots are among your most potent allies when it comes to protecting your heart. That's important because blood sugar problems raise your risk of heart disease.

Makes 6 servings

1 pound large carrots, peeled and cut into long, thin slices

¼ teaspoon salt

1½ teaspoons olive oil

1 teaspoon minced fresh rosemary leaves or ½ teaspoon dried, crumbled

1. Preheat the oven to 400°F.

2. Mound the carrot slices on a baking sheet. Sprinkle with the salt and drizzle with the oil. Gently toss. Spread them out on the sheet into a single layer.

3. Stir in the rosemary. Roast until crisp-tender and lightly browned in spots, 7 to 10 minutes.

PER SERVING **Nutrition info:** 44 calories, 1 g protein, 8 g carbohydrate, 1 g total fat, 0 g saturated fat, 0 mg cholesterol, 2 g fiber, 136 mg sodium

2 Day Diabetes Diet exchanges: 1 vegetable

Baked Sweet Potato "Fries"

Many people buy frozen, premade fries (and Ian's and Alexa varieties are perfectly acceptable options for this plan). Still, these delights are actually very easy to make at home. And unlike the fried version, they are light on calories but still high on satisfaction.

Makes 4 servings

1 pound sweet potatoes, peeled and cut into ½"-thick "fries"

1 tablespoon vegetable oil

¼ teaspoon salt

¼ teaspoon ground black pepper

1. Preheat the oven to 425°F. Lightly coat a baking sheet with cooking spray.

2. In a large bowl, combine the sweet potatoes, oil, salt, and pepper. Toss to coat. Spread the fries in a single layer on the baking sheet.

3. Bake for 10 minutes. Turn the fries over. Continue baking until they are tender and lightly browned, about 10 minutes longer.

PER SERVING **Nutrition info:** 102 calories, 2 g protein, 17 g carbohydrate, 4 g total fat, 0 g saturated fat, 0 mg cholesterol, 3g fiber, 152 mg sodium

2 Day Diabetes Diet exchanges: 1 starch, 1 fat

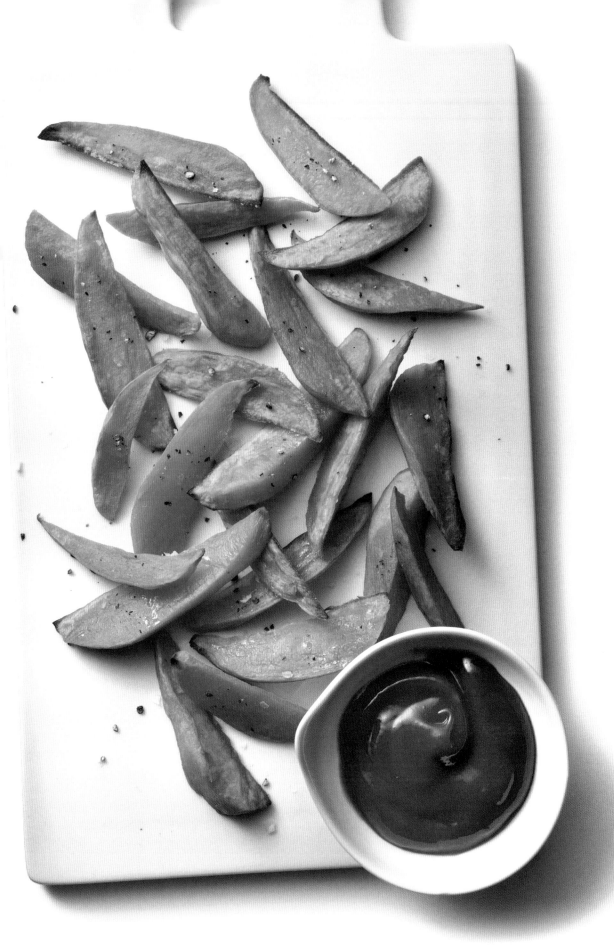

Baked Tomato

At only 76 calories per serving, this simple recipe is a great option for Power Burn Days. On Nourishment Days, you can top the tomatoes with part-skim mozzarella cheese for an extra serving of protein!

Makes 1 serving

1   medium tomato, sliced horizontally in half

2   tablespoons grated low-fat Parmesan cheese

1   teaspoon dried oregano

Salt to taste

Ground black pepper to taste

Preheat the oven to 450°F. Place the tomato halves cut side up on a baking sheet and spray the cut sides with cooking spray. Top the tomatoes with the Parmesan cheese, oregano, and salt and pepper to taste. Bake for 15 minutes.

PER SERVING **Nutrition info:** 76 calories, 6 g protein, 7 g carbohydrate, 3 g total fat, 2 g saturated fat, 8 mg cholesterol, 2 g fiber, 435 mg sodium

2 Day Diabetes Diet exchanges: 1 vegetable, 1 oz protein

Mashed Cauliflower

Mashed potatoes digest quickly, causing massive blood sugar spikes. Mashed cauliflower, on the other hand, tastes almost as creamy, but with much less of a carb load. Eat them without guilt.

Makes 2 servings

2   cups fresh cauliflower, steamed

2   tablespoons whipped butter or light trans-fat-free margarine

¼   teaspoon salt

1   teaspoon ground black pepper

Steam the cauliflower until tender. Place the cauliflower, butter or margarine, salt, and pepper in a blender or food processor. Blend on high until smooth. Serve warm.

PER SERVING **Nutrition info:** 107 calories, 2 g protein, 5 g carbohydrate, 9 g total fat, 6 g saturated fat, 25 mg cholesterol, 3 g fiber, 996 mg sodium

2 Day Diabetes Diet exchanges: 1 vegetable, 1 fat

Pineapple Coleslaw

Coleslaw is easier to make than most people think, especially if you start with a prepared mix. The shredded cabbage can help you drop your cholesterol level and reduce your risk for cancer. Along with spinach, it's one type of green that has been shown to reduce the risk for diabetes, too.

Makes 8 servings

1 bag coleslaw mix

1 green bell pepper, finely chopped

1 can (20 ounces) unsweetened crushed pineapple

2 tablespoons fat-free mayonnaise

1 tablespoon wine vinegar

1 teaspoon Dijon or honey mustard

2 packets Splenda or Equal sweetener

Salt and freshly ground black pepper, to taste

1. Combine the coleslaw mix, green pepper, and pineapple (with liquid) in a large bowl.

2. Stir together the mayonnaise, vinegar, mustard, sweetener, salt, and pepper in a small bowl. Add to the cabbage mixture and stir well to combine. Chill for several hours or overnight. Mix well before serving.

PER SERVING **Nutrition info:** 60 calories, 1 g protein, 12 g carbohydrate, 0 g total fat, 0 g saturated fat, 0 mg cholesterol, 2 g fiber, 10 mg sodium

2 Day Diabetes Diet exchanges: 1 vegetable, ½ fruit

Bulgur with Spring Vegetables

Made from wheat berries, this side takes only 20 to 30 minutes to cook—much less time than other whole grains such as brown rice. It's also loaded with fiber and digests slowly, providing a slow, even rise in blood sugar levels.

Makes 6 servings

1 ¼   cups bulgur

3 ½   cups boiling water

2   tablespoons olive oil, divided

3   tablespoons freshly squeezed lemon juice

⅛   teaspoon salt

½   teaspoon ground black pepper

2   leeks, halved lengthwise and cut crosswise into 1" pieces

2   cloves garlic, minced

12   asparagus spears, cut into 2" lengths

1   cup frozen peas

¼   cup chopped fresh mint

1. In a large heatproof bowl, combine the bulgur and boiling water. Let stand until the bulgur is tender, about 30 minutes, stirring after 15 minutes. Drain the bulgur in a large fine-meshed sieve to get rid of any remaining liquid.

2. In a large bowl, whisk together 1 tablespoon of the oil and the lemon juice, salt, and pepper. Add the drained bulgur and fluff with a fork.

3. In a medium skillet over low heat, heat the remaining 1 tablespoon oil. Add the leeks and garlic to the skillet and cook until the leeks are tender, about 5 minutes. Transfer to the bowl with the bulgur.

4. In a steamer set over boiling water, steam the asparagus until tender, about 4 minutes. Add the peas during the final 30 seconds of steaming. Add the vegetables to the bowl of bulgur, along with the mint, and toss to combine. Serve at room temperature or chilled.

PER SERVING **Nutrition info:** 188 calories, 6 g protein, 32 g carbohydrate, 5 g total fat, 0.5 g saturated fat, 0 mg cholesterol, 8 g fiber, 330 mg sodium

2 Day Diabetes Diet exchanges: 1 vegetable, 1 starch, 1 fat

Tabbouleh

This colorful and healthful Middle Eastern dish can be refrigerated for up to 4 days. If you use radishes, add them just before serving.

Makes 4 servings

1	cup boiling water
¾	cup bulgur
1	medium red onion, chopped (1 cup)
1	medium tomato, coarsely chopped, with juice (1 cup)
½	cucumber, seeded and coarsely chopped (½ cup)
4	large radishes, slivered (optional)
1	cup coarsely chopped flat-leaf parsley
2	tablespoons minced fresh mint or 2 teaspoons mint flakes, crumbled
1	tablespoon olive oil or canola oil
1	teaspoon lemon zest
4	tablespoons lemon juice
¾	teaspoon salt
8	to 10 drops hot red-pepper sauce

1. In a large heatproof serving bowl, pour 1 cup of boiling water over the bulgur and let stand for 20 minutes or until the water is absorbed. Meanwhile, in a small bowl, pour just enough boiling water over the onion to cover and let stand for 10 minutes. Drain.

2. Add the onion, tomato, cucumber, radishes (if using), parsley, mint, oil, lemon zest, lemon juice, salt, and red-pepper sauce to the bulgur. Toss until well combined. Refrigerate, covered, for 6 hours or until chilled. Serve cold or at room temperature.

PER SERVING **Nutrition info:** 153 calories, 5 g protein, 28 g carbohydrate, 4 g total fat, 1 g saturated fat, 0 mg cholesterol, 8 g fiber, 418 mg sodium

2 Day Diabetes Diet exchanges: 1 vegetable, 1 starch, 1 fat

Tex-Mex Red Beans

Beans make for an incredibly filling side dish or meal unto themselves. To turn this recipe into a Nourishment Day meal, use the beans as a filling for whole-grain enchiladas. Or create a taco salad.

Makes 6 servings

1 cup dried red kidney beans

2 quarts water

2 tablespoons olive oil or canola oil

2 onions, coarsely chopped

2 cloves garlic, finely chopped

2 red or green bell peppers, chopped

1 can (14 ounces) crushed tomatoes

1 bay leaf

¼ teaspoon dried thyme

⅛ teaspoon ground cumin

⅛ teaspoon salt

⅛ teaspoon ground black pepper

1 cup vegetable stock

1. Place the beans in a medium bowl. Add enough cold water to cover and let stand for 8 hours. Drain. In a large pot, boil the beans in the 2 quarts water for 10 minutes, then turn down the heat and simmer for 45 minutes. Drain.

2. In a Dutch oven, heat the oil. Sauté the onions and garlic, stirring, for 5 minutes. Add the bell peppers and sauté for 5 minutes longer.

3. Add the tomatoes, bay leaf, thyme, cumin, salt, and black pepper, stir, and bring to a boil. Stir in the beans and stock. Simmer, partially covered, for 20 minutes. Discard the bay leaf before serving.

PER SERVING **Nutrition info:** 201 calories, 10 g protein, 32 g carbohydrate, 5 g total fat, 1 g saturated fat, 9 mg cholesterol, 10 g fiber, 131 mg sodium

2 Day Diabetes Diet exchanges: 1 vegetable, 1 starch, 1 oz protein, 1 fat

Crispy Cheese Chips

There's no need to resort to store-bought cheese chips when you can make this healthier version at home.

Makes 2 servings

28" whole-wheat tortillas
2 tablespoons olive oil
1 clove garlic, minced
½ teaspoon dried basil
¼ cup Parmesan cheese

1. Preheat the oven to 350°F. Cut the tortillas into 8 triangle-shaped wedges.

2. Coat a baking sheet with cooking spray.

3. In a small bowl, combine the olive oil, garlic, and basil. Brush this mixture over each of the tortilla wedges. Sprinkle Parmesan cheese over all the wedges.

4. Bake for 8 to 9 minutes, or until toasted.

PER SERVING **Nutrition info:** 148 calories, 4.5 g protein, 10 g carbohydrate, 10 g total fat, 2.5 g saturated fat, 7.5 mg cholesterol, 0.5 g fiber, 211 mg sodium

2 Day Diabetes Diet exchanges: 1 starch, 1 oz protein, 3 fat

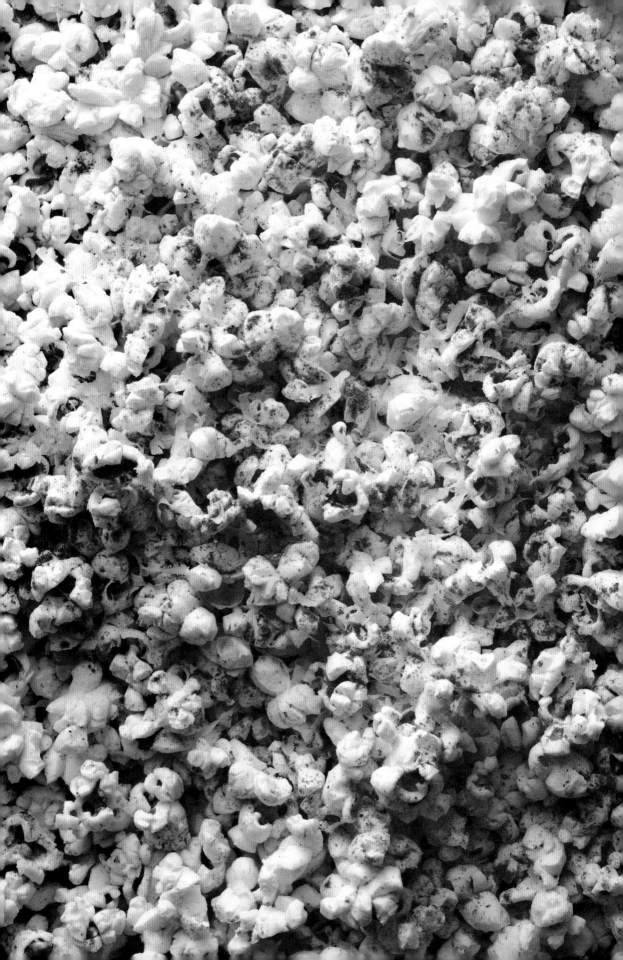

Chili Popcorn

To cut back on the saturated fat from butter and some of the salt, this tasty treat uses the spicy flavors of paprika and chili powder.

Makes 10 servings (1 cup each)

1   teaspoon paprika

½   teaspoon chili powder

¼   teaspoon salt

⅛   teaspoon garlic powder

Pinch of cayenne pepper, or to taste

1   tablespoon grated Parmesan cheese

10   cups popped corn made without salt or oil

Butter-flavored cooking spray (optional)

1. Preheat the oven to 350°F. In a small bowl, combine the paprika, chili powder, salt, garlic powder, cayenne pepper, and Parmesan cheese.

2. Spread the popcorn in an even layer on 2 large baking sheets and coat lightly with the cooking spray, if using, or with water from a spray bottle. With a fork, sprinkle the seasonings over the popcorn and toss the popcorn to coat.

3. Bake for 5 to 10 minutes or until crisp. Serve immediately or store in an airtight container.

PER SERVING **Nutrition info:** 29 calories, 1 g protein, 5 g carbohydrate, 0 g total fat, 0 g saturated fat, 0 mg cholesterol, 0 g fiber, 66 mg sodium

2 Day Diabetes Diet exchanges: ⅓ starch

Yogurt Fruit Dip

This recipe makes a great dip for sliced fruit. It's a sweet treat that works as a side dish as well as a snack.

Makes 1 serving

- 1 tablespoon vanilla extract
- 1 tablespoon ground cinnamon
- 1 packet artificial sweetener (optional)
- 1 cup 2% plain Greek yogurt

Blend the vanilla, cinnamon, and sweetener (if desired) into the yogurt. Serve chilled.

PER SERVING **Nutrition info:** 199 calories, 12 g protein, 24 g carbohydrate, 4 g total fat, 2 g saturated fat, 14 mg cholesterol, 4 g fiber, 160 mg sodium

2 Day Diabetes Diet exchanges: 1 dairy

Yogurt Vegetable Dip

Usually dip is loaded with fat and calories. This version leans on spices and Greek yogurt for its naturally low-calorie creaminess. Quadruple the recipe to serve it with sliced veggies at your next get-together. No one will be the wiser.

Makes 1 serving

- 1 cup 2% plain Greek yogurt
- ½ teaspoon dried dill
- ¼ teaspoon ground white pepper

Salt to taste

In a small bowl, mix the yogurt, dill, pepper, and salt to form a creamy vegetable dip. Serve chilled.

PER SERVING **Nutrition info:** 170 calories, 23 g protein, 9 g carbohydrate, 4.5 g total fat, 3 g saturated fat, 12 mg cholesterol, 0 g fiber, 191 mg sodium

2 Day Diabetes Diet exchanges: 1 dairy

Cherry-Turmeric Yogurt

This unusual flavor combo is great if you suffer from digestive ills. Turmeric has been shown to reduce symptoms of gas and bloating, and yogurt contains beneficial bacteria shown to heal the digestive tract.

Makes 1 serving

1   teaspoon ground turmeric

1   cup 2% plain Greek yogurt

1   teaspoon vanilla extract (optional)

½   teaspoon calorie-free sweetener (optional)

2   tablespoons dried tart cherries

Stir the turmeric into the yogurt until fully dissolved. If desired, flavor the yogurt with the vanilla and calorie-free sweetener. Top with the tart cherries and enjoy.

PER SERVING **Nutrition info:** 168 calories, 13 g protein, 21 g carbohydrate, 4 g total fat, 2 g saturated fat, 14 mg cholesterol, 1 g fiber, 162 mg sodium

2 Day Diabetes Diet exchanges: 1 fruit, 1 dairy

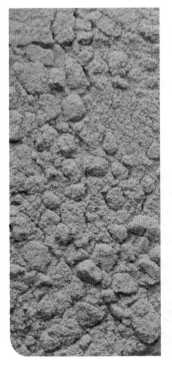

SUPERFOOD SPOTLIGHT: Turmeric

Turmeric is a spice that may have been protecting the health of an entire Indian subcontinent for about 5,000 years. While the traditional Indian diet with white rice and flour breads has a lot of rapidly digested carbs that would ordinarily raise blood sugar dramatically, the presence of turmeric—the yellow spice that lends its color to many curry dishes—helps to manage the potent impact on blood sugar. Curcumin, the active ingredient in turmeric, is the compound believed to regulate fat metabolism in the body. Curcumin acts directly on fat cells, pancreatic cells, kidney cells, and muscle cells, dampening inflammation and blocking the nefarious activities of cancer-causing tumor necrosis factor and interleukin-6. Experts believe the combined action of all of these factors together gives curcumin the power to reverse insulin resistance, high blood sugar and high cholesterol, and other symptoms linked to obesity. You don't have to love Indian food to get your turmeric—you can throw it into your eggs in the morning, or you can sprinkle it on your salads or yogurt dips in the afternoon or your cauliflower at dinner and over baked apples for dessert.

Bouillon Fruit Stew

This sweet, filling soup is just what you need to go the distance on your Power Burn Days.

Makes 2 servings

2   cups water, divided

1¾ cups frozen strawberries, thawed

¼   cup orange juice

2   vegetable bouillon cubes

1. In a blender or food processor, place 1 cup of the water and all of the strawberries. Blend until pureed and smooth.

2. In a large pot, bring the remaining 1 cup water and the orange juice to a boil. Add the bouillon cubes and stir until dissolved.

3. Reduce the heat to a simmer and add the pureed berries. Stir for 2 minutes, or until the mixture is adequately blended.

4. Remove from the heat and chill in the refrigerator for 3 hours. Serve chilled.

PER SERVING **Nutrition info:** 34 calories, 0.5 g protein, 8 g carbohydrate, 0 g total fat, 0 g saturated fat, 0 mg cholesterol, 1 g fiber, 30 mg sodium

2 Day Diabetes Diet exchanges: ½ fruit, 8 oz bouillon

Apple-Cinnamon Smoothie

Why consume all that sugar at the bottom of a yogurt cup when you can make your own just-as-delicious version with fewer calories?

Makes 1 serving

1   cup 2% plain yogurt (regular or Greek)

½   cup unsweetened applesauce

1   tablespoon vanilla extract

1   teaspoon ground cinnamon

½   cup ice

In a blender, combine the yogurt, applesauce, vanilla, cinnamon, and ice. Blend on high for 1 minute or until the desired consistency is reached. Serve cold.

PER SERVING **Nutrition info:** 232 calories, 12 g protein, 32 g carbohydrate, 4 g total fat, 2 g saturated fat, 14 mg cholesterol, 2 g fiber, 162 mg sodium

2 Day Diabetes Diet exchanges: 1 fruit, 1 dairy

Black Cherry Smoothie

Both blackberries and cherries are rich in plant nutrients that help to repair your cells. Cherries, in particular, contain many powerful compounds that are thought to fend off cancer, arthritis, and premature aging. They might even reduce the incidence of migraines.

Makes 1 serving

1 cup 2% plain yogurt (regular or Greek)

½ cup blackberries, fresh or frozen

5 cherries

½ cup ice

In a blender, combine the yogurt, blackberries, cherries, and ice. Blend on high for 1 minute or until the desired consistency is reached. Serve cold.

PER SERVING **Nutrition info:** 264 calories, 14 g protein, 45 g carbohydrate, 5 g total fat, 2 g saturated fat, 14 mg cholesterol, 8 g fiber, 161 mg sodium

2 Day Diabetes Diet exchanges: 1 fruit, 1 dairy

Blueberry Smoothie

This morning delight brings you one of your superfoods in an easy-to-consume package.

Makes 1 serving

1 cup 2% plain yogurt (regular or Greek)

1 cup fresh or frozen blueberries

1 tablespoon vanilla extract

½ cup ice

In a blender, combine the yogurt, blueberries, vanilla, and ice. Blend on high for 1 minute or until the desired consistency is reached. Serve cold.

PER SERVING **Nutrition info:** 259 calories, 13 g protein, 37 g carbohydrate, 5 g total fat, 2 g saturated fat, 14 mg cholesterol, 4 g fiber, 161 mg sodium

2 Day Diabetes Diet exchanges: 1 fruit, 1 dairy

Mango Smoothie

To make the prep work easier for this delicious smoothie, keep frozen mango chunks on hand. Toss them straight into the blender and then omit the ice.

Makes 1 serving

1 cup 2% plain yogurt (regular or Greek)

½ cup chopped mango

1 teaspoon ground psyllium husk

1 packet artificial sweetener (optional)

½ cup ice

In a blender, combine the yogurt, mango, psyllium, sweetener (if using), and ice. Blend on high for 1 minute or until the desired consistency is reached. Serve cold.

PER SERVING **Nutrition info:** 202 calories, 13 g protein, 31 g carbohydrate, 4 g total fat, 2 g saturated fat, 14 mg cholesterol, 3 g fiber, 161 mg sodium

2 Day Diabetes Diet exchanges: 1 fruit, 1 dairy

Peach Crisp

The good fats in the walnuts, the fiber in the oats, and the nutrients in the peaches make this treat a health star.

Makes 9 servings

4   cups sliced fresh or frozen peaches

¾   cup Splenda sweetener

1   teaspoon ground cinnamon

½   cup old-fashioned oats

2   tablespoons chopped walnuts

½   cup graham cracker crumbs

½   cup brown sugar

2   tablespoons light tub margarine

1. Preheat the oven to 350°F.

2. Place the peaches in an 8" x 8" baking dish and sprinkle them with the sweetener and cinnamon.

3. For the topping, stir together the oats, walnuts, graham cracker crumbs, and brown sugar in a medium bowl. Blend in the margarine. Scatter the oat mixture over the peaches and bake until crisp on top, about 45 minutes.

4. For an even quicker version of Peach Crisp, top with peaches-and-cream instant oatmeal instead of making the topping.

PER SERVING **Nutrition info:** 140 calories, 2 g protein, 27 g carbohydrate, 3 g total fat, 1 g saturated fat, 0 mg cholesterol, 2 g fiber, 75 mg sodium

2 Day Diabetes Diet exchanges: ½ fruit, 1 ¼ starch

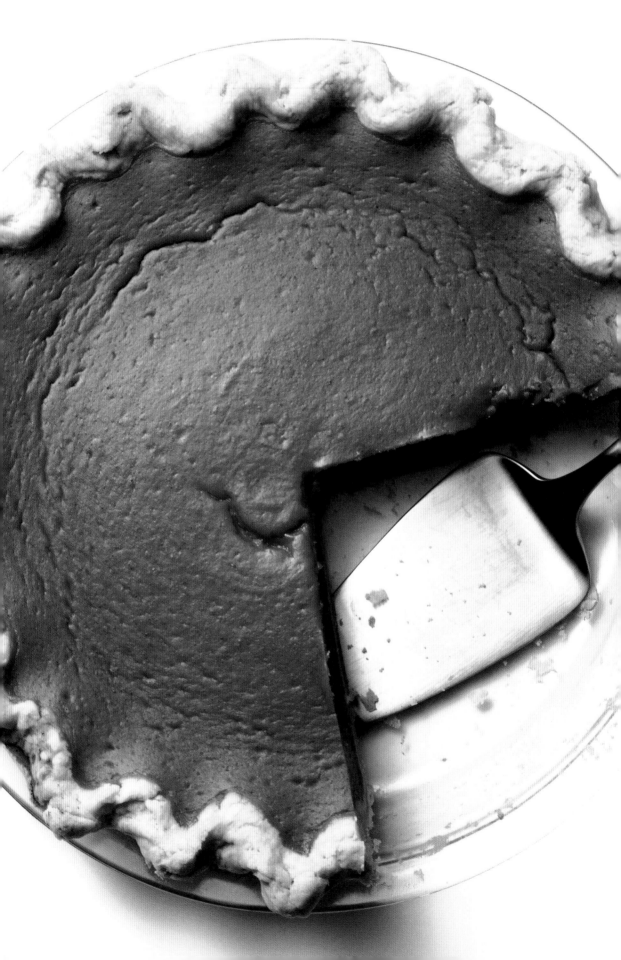

Pumpkin Pie

Did you think you'd have to go off the plan during Thanksgiving?
Think again. This pumpkin pie recipe allows you to indulge and stay
true to the plan.

Makes 8 servings

For the crust:

1 cup all-purpose flour

½ teaspoon salt

6 tablespoons light stick margarine, chilled

2–3 tablespoons ice water

For the sauce:

1 can (16 ounces) pumpkin

1 can (12 ounces) fat-free evaporated milk

4 egg whites

18 packets (¾ cup) Equal sweetener

Spoonful of Splenda sweetener

¼ teaspoon salt

1 teaspoon ground cinnamon

½ teaspoon ground ginger

⅓ teaspoon ground cloves

1. Preheat the oven to 425°F.

2. To make the crust: Stir together the flour and salt in a medium bowl. Cut in the margarine. Gradually add the water and stir until moistened. Shape into a ball and roll into a 10" circle. Place in a 9" pie pan and crimp the edges.

3. To make the filling: Beat the pumpkin, milk, and egg whites with an electric mixer in a medium bowl. Add the Equal sweetener, Splenda sweetener, salt, cinnamon, ginger, and cloves and beat until combined.

4. Pour the filling into the crust and bake for 15 minutes, then reduce the heat to 350°F and bake for about 40 minutes longer. Cool on a wire rack.

PER SERVING **Nutrition info:** 155 calories, 7 g protein, 22 g carbohydrate, 5 g total fat, 1 g saturated fat, 0 mg cholesterol, 2 g fiber, 380 mg sodium

2 Day Diabetes Diet exchanges: 1 starch, ¼ protein, 1 fat

Chocolate-Banana Pudding Parfait

Pudding is one of those creamy delights that many people just can't live without. Here's good news: You don't have to live without it! A sugar-free mix and fat-free milk and topping render this pudding completely diet friendly.

Makes 4 servings

1 package (1.4 ounces) sugar-free chocolate pudding

2 cups fat-free milk

1 banana, sliced

4 ounces fat-free or light whipped topping

1 teaspoon shaved chocolate

1. Make the pudding according to package directions, using the fat-free milk. Layer the pudding with the banana slices in 4 parfait glasses.

2. Add a dollop of the whipped topping, sprinkle with the shaved chocolate, and serve.

PER SERVING Nutrition info: 150 calories, 5 g protein, 30 g carbohydrate, 0 g total fat, 0 g saturated fat, 3 mg cholesterol, 0 g fiber, 395 mg sodium

2 Day Diabetes Diet exchanges: ½ fruit, ½ starch, ½ dairy

Marble Cheesecake

Cheesecake? In a diet book!?! Yes, indeed. This cheesecake recipe leans on silken tofu and low-fat and fat-free ingredients to cut calories without sacrificing satisfaction. Even so, it's still relatively rich in starch and calories, so include it with a starchless, low-fat dinner and reserve it as an occasional (not everyday) delight.

Makes 12 servings

6   whole low-fat honey graham crackers

½   cup toasted wheat germ

1   tablespoon + 1 cup sugar

2   tablespoons extra-light olive oil

1   container (19 ounces) silken tofu, well drained

1   pound fat-free cream cheese

3   tablespoons flour

1   large egg + 2 large egg whites

1   teaspoon vanilla

¼   cup chocolate syrup

1. Preheat the oven to 350°F. Combine the graham crackers, wheat germ, and 1 tablespoon sugar in a food processor and process to fine crumbs. Add the oil and process until moistened. Place the mixture in a 9" springform pan and press it into the bottom and partway up the sides. Bake until set, about 10 minutes.

2. Add the drained tofu, remaining 1 cup sugar, cream cheese, flour, whole egg, egg whites, and vanilla to the food processor (no need to clean the bowl) and process until smooth and well blended.

3. Measure out 1 cup of the tofu mixture, place it in a small bowl, and stir in the chocolate syrup. Pour the remaining plain tofu mixture into the crust in the springform pan.

4. Pour the chocolate mixture in a ring on top of the batter and swirl it in with a knife. Bake for 45 minutes. Turn off the oven and leave the cheesecake in the oven 45 minutes longer, undisturbed. Cool to room temperature before chilling overnight.

PER SERVING **Nutrition info:** 225 calories, 11 g protein, 35 g carbohydrate, 5 g total fat, 1 g saturated fat, 21 mg cholesterol, 1 g fiber, 245 mg sodium

2 Day Diabetes Diet exchanges: 2 starch, 1 ½ oz protein, 1 fat

CHAPTER 10

The 2 Day Diabetes Diet
Tension Taming Plan

Stress can worsen diabetes and make it harder to lose weight. Four simple exercises help you relax and resist food cravings.

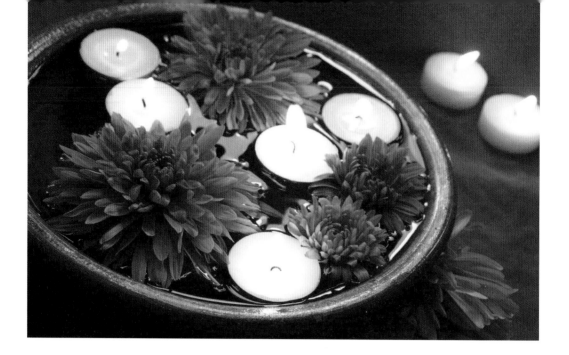

When most people think about what it takes to turn around blood sugar problems, relaxation is probably the last thing that comes to mind.

Yet relaxation is actually vitally important for your success. Why? Stress can complicate diabetes by distracting you from what you need to do to keep it under control. Think about it: When you are feeling harried, are you generally on top of your self-care game? For most people, the answer is no. As soon as life gets complicated, they start eating poorly, skipping exercise sessions, and forgetting to test their blood sugar.

Stress can also worsen diabetes directly. As we mentioned earlier, when levels of the stress hormone cortisol rise, your liver dumps glucose into your bloodstream in an attempt to make fuel easily available for cells. In people with diabetes, however, the fight-or-flight response works more like a bathtub that drains into a water pipe that's clogged up with old soap scum. Turn on the faucet in such a bathtub and water fills the tub, but it doesn't drain back out very quickly. This is exactly what happens inside the pipes that make up your arteries. The liver turns on the glucose faucet, but, because of insulin resistance, glucose doesn't drain out of the bloodstream and into hungry cells as it should. So every time your liver turns on the faucet, your blood glucose readings climb, and they stay elevated longer than needed.

Stress can also interfere with your efforts to drop pounds. What's the first food that comes to mind when you are under stress? We're guessing it's not broccoli or kale, but rather something more like cookies, chips, or fries. That's because rises in cortisol are designed to trigger our appetites for high-calorie foods. After all, our bodies evolved to face stressors like dangerous wild animals. Fending off such a stressor resulted in lots of burned energy—energy that needed to be replaced. In modern times, however, most stressors don't burn many, if any, calories. Sitting in traffic? Worrying about finishing a report by a given deadline? Steaming over that condescending remark? Not many calories burned, right? Yet your body doesn't know the difference, so now you're hungry even though your cells don't need more calories.

Even if you don't give in to stress-induced cravings, stress can make you feel too tired to cook or shop, causing you to reach for fast calories from packaged foods or fast food.

Ready to tame that tension? We sure hope so.

Your Power-Burning Ally

As we've mentioned, research shows that cultivating calm also gives your weight-loss and blood sugar–control efforts a powerful boost. That makes Tension Tamers great for every day of the week, but they are especially important on Power Burn Days. On your Power Burn Days, you're working hard to stay true to the plan. This can create tension in and of itself, especially in the beginning as you are getting used to the diet. Your Tension Tamers will help you focus less on food and more on a general state of calm. Consider doing a Tension Tamer:

FAQ: IF I'M PRETTY CHILL, DO I NEED TO DO TENSION TAMERS?

Tension Tamers are good for everyone, and we highly recommend them. That said, if you'd like some firsthand evidence for whether stress is affecting your blood sugar, here's a simple way to find out. On a scale of 1 to 10, jot down your level of stress and then check your glucose levels. Do this every day for a couple weeks, keeping a record of your glucose readings and the corresponding amount of stress. Then look over your written record and see if there's a pattern. Chances are, you'll be able to see that higher stress numbers result in higher blood sugar numbers.

- ► Whenever you feel tempted to eat more than what's on your plate
- ► Whenever you feel tempted to eat something that you didn't plan to eat
- ► Before bed, to encourage a more restful sleep
- ► Before meals, so you can take that first bite with a more present mind
- ► Whenever you feel tense

Tension Tamers are optional, but we recommend you set a goal to do at least one on your Power Burn Days. Once you get the hang of it, add another. They're short enough that you could easily do all four each day. (And while we encourage you to do them on your Power Burn Days, there's no reason you can't do them every day, if you choose.)

Choose the Belly-Breathing Exercise or the Sighing Exercise (it also uses breath to relax you) when you've got just a few minutes, the Muscle Relaxation Technique or Limb Relaxation Exercise when you've got about 10 minutes. The Sighing Exercise is a great choice to start your day, and the Muscle Relaxation Technique is delicious to do before bed. Sneak the Belly-Breathing Exercise and the Limb Relaxation Exercise into your day at midmorning and midafternoon (or as soon as you arrive home from work).

Sighing Exercise

1. Sit or stand with your back straight and your hands at your sides or resting on your knees. Let the air rush out of your lungs as if you were deeply relieved that a stressful event has passed (even if it hasn't).
2. Forget about how you're breathing in for a moment. Just take another breath naturally, and let it rush out again.
3. Repeat 10 times for a total of 12 sighs. By the time you've finished, it won't feel like you're sighing anymore. Instead, you'll be breathing deeply.

Belly-Breathing Exercise

1. Find a quiet place, and sit comfortably with your back straight against the back of a chair. Place one hand on your chest and the other on your stomach, then breathe normally. Pay attention to which hand moves the most as you inhale and exhale. If it's the one on your chest, the lower areas of your lungs are not filling with air.

2. Take in a deep breath through your nose. Inhale slowly so you can't hear your breathing; if the rush of air makes a noise, you're inhaling too quickly. Fill the bottom sections of your lungs first so your diaphragm pushes the hand on your stomach outward. Continue to inhale until you fill the upper parts of your lungs, making the hand on your chest rise slightly.

3. Hold your breath for a moment, and think of the word relax. Exhale slowly and naturally (it's okay if you can hear the air escaping). Continue breathing in and out slowly for several minutes.

> **Tension Tamers are especially important on Power Burn days.**

Muscle Relaxation Technique

1. Lie down or sit in a comfortable chair that supports your head. Close your eyes, and mentally scan your body for places that feel tense.

2. Working slowly from your feet to your head, clench each muscle area as tightly as you can and hold for 5 seconds. Take about 20 seconds to gradually release the tension, consciously relaxing your muscles as much as possible, then move on to the next area.

3. Silently repeat a soothing thought, such as "I am totally calm" or "Goodbye, tension" as you work your way up to your forehead.

Limb Relaxation Exercise

Perform this exercise in a quiet room. You can sit in a comfortable chair that supports your head, back, and arms, or you can sit slightly stooped on a stool, with your arms resting on your thighs and your hands hanging loosely between your knees. After you're settled into position with your eyes closed, do the following sequence:

1. Concentrate your attention on your dominant arm, usually the right. Slowly repeat, "My right arm is heavy" in your mind, and imagine the arm actually becoming heavier. Pause after the statement, repeating it four times.

2. Do the same with your left arm.

3. Next, repeat the exercise using the words, "Both my arms are heavy."

4. Concentrate on your right leg, and slowly repeat, "My right leg is heavy" four times.

5. Do the same with your left leg, then both legs.

6. Repeat the exercise, but this time use the word warm instead of heavy, and imagine your limbs becoming warmer. Once you're used to this technique, you can do another exercise in which you imagine your limbs becoming heavier and warmer at the same time. It's possible that you'll enter a trancelike state—which is fine. When you're finished with the exercise, simply mark its completion by telling yourself, "When I open my eyes, I will be refreshed and alert."

More Ways to Tame Tension

In addition to the exercises we just suggested, you can tame tension even more by doing the following:

Be social. Sometimes when the pressure's on, we tend to isolate ourselves. But contact with friends and family is often an effective way to take your mind off your troubles. A chat with a buddy can make you feel less alone, and a bit of moral support from a friend can go a long way. If you're busy, a short phone call or e-mail could be enough to keep you feeling connected. Also try doing volunteer work, which can strengthen your connection to your community.

Simplify. A cluttered life can add stress to your day in countless ways. When you're always scrambling to find the car keys or you're not sure which bills have been paid because the stack of mail is a mess . . . well, you get the idea. The key to clearing out clutter is to start small. Pick one room, one shelf, one drawer. Separate what you really need from what you can toss out or donate. If the job seems too overwhelming, consider hiring a professional organizer to get you started.

Do one thing at a time. Multitasking is so old-fashioned. New research shows that trying to do many things at once—watching TV while you read your e-mail, check your phone messages, and surf the Net— makes it harder to concentrate. You end up taking more time to finish your tasks, adding to your stress and workload. Doing one thing at a time, however, can put you in a zone, with total concentration on what you're doing and a fulfilling sense of accomplishment. Try it!

Try something new. In some ways, this is a good time to be stressed: There are more options out there for stress management than ever before. Whether it's yoga, meditation, tai chi, mindfulness, or one of the many other activities available to help manage stress, there's almost certainly something that will work for you.

Schedule some daily downtime. Every day, no matter how busy you may be, give yourself at least 10 to 20 minutes of quiet reflection. Use the time to listen to relaxing music, breathe deeply, and relax your tense muscles. Consider doing your Tension Tamers during this time.

Laugh! Sometimes laughter really is the best medicine, and science shows that whatever makes you laugh also does good things for your body. A good laugh brings oxygen to your heart, lungs, and muscles, it stimulates circulation, aids muscle relaxation, and releases natural "feel-good" hormones called endorphins. Studies also show that over time, laughter boosts your immune system, eases pain, and enhances social connections with other people. So spend time with those friends who always have you chortling. Find time to see a funny movie, or watch the Internet videos or TV comedies that leave you laughing. Keep a book by your favorite comedian or humorist handy, so you can dip into it when you need a laugh.

CHAPTER 11

The 2 Day Diabetes Diet Exercise Plan

Exercise reduces insulin resistance, melts belly fat, and gets you to your goal weight faster. This easy three-step plan is the perfect recipe for improved health and vitality.

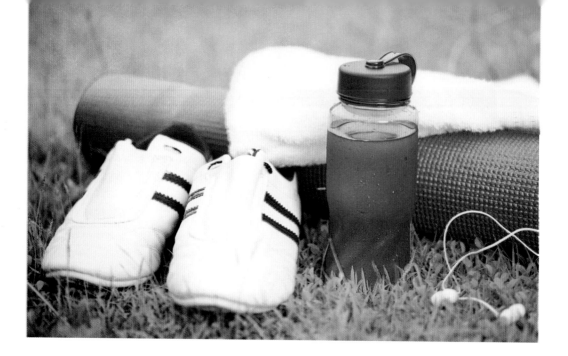

The 2 plus 5 eating approach—with its emphasis on blood sugar-friendly superfoods—is so effective that it's really all you need to achieve lasting success. Just by following the meal plans, food options, and advice in Levels 1, 2, and 3 of the plan you'll be well on your way to reversing your blood sugar problems and dropping those stubborn pounds for good.

That said, we highly encourage you to give the 2 Day Diabetes Diet's exercise plan a try. We worked hard to ensure that this plan was not only effective for people with diabetes or who are prone to developing it, but also realistic. If you are rushed for time, a beginner, or someone who claims to be "allergic to exercise," this plan just might be the one that makes you an exercise convert.

The 2 Day Diabetes Diet exercise plan includes an easy walking program plus a quick strength-building routine. It doesn't take much time or require you to buy any special equipment. If you've got sneakers or walking shoes, a towel, comfortable clothing, and a chair or kitchen counter to use for some of the strength moves, you're good to go.

If you're already active—you're a dedicated walker, an active gardener or golfer, you go to the gym or ride a bike, for example—then just keep up the good work by continuing what you are already doing so successfully. If you are not already active, the 2 Day Diabetes Diet's plan is a great way to start. You'll start very slowly on this plan, with just 10 minutes of walking (at your own pace) 3 days a week. Gradually, you'll add more minutes and more steps. The plan's safe, easy, specially designed strength-training routine will help you build more muscle in just two 20-minute sessions per week. For convenience, you can even split the strength-training routine into three mini workouts that take just 6 to 7 minutes apiece—something you can fit into your busiest day.

Doable? You bet.

10 Reasons to Say "Yes" to Exercise

If you opt in to the 2 Day Diabetes Diet exercise plan, you can expect to reap many, many benefits. Among them, you'll:

Get to your goal faster. Study after study shows that regular physical activity can help you to burn more calories, torch more body fat (especially belly fat), reduce your blood sugar levels, and build more sexy, sugar-sipping muscle. The results will amaze you. In a 2011 study from Seattle's Fred Hutchinson Cancer Research Center, women who followed a healthy, reduced-calorie diet and exercised regularly lost an average of 19.8 pounds in a year. In contrast, those who only exercised lost an average of 4.4 pounds and those who only dieted lost 15.8 pounds.[1]

Stay at your goal for life. Exercise also helps you keep weight off—a major challenge once you've lost those extra pounds. In one 2010 study from the Arizona Cancer Center, women who did muscle-building moves on a regular basis were 22 percent less likely to put on pounds and body fat than women who didn't strength-train.[2]

Manage blood sugar more easily. Think of activity as a sponge that helps soak up excess sugar that's circulating

EXERCISE EARLY, EAT LESS

Want to trim your appetite and your figure? Move your body—and also, possibly, your workout. New research out of Brigham Young University in Salt Lake City showed that 45 minutes of moderate to vigorous exercise in the morning reduced the brain's interest in food. The study authors measured the neural activity of 35 women while they viewed food images, following both a morning of exercise and a morning without exercise. And they found that the women's "attentional response" to the pics decreased after the brisk workout.

around your system. When muscles contract, your body sends out armies of sugar-moving proteins called GLUT-4 transporters that carry sugar molecules from your bloodstream into your cells. This process doesn't rely on insulin (the hormone that tells cells to let blood sugar in). And the benefits can last for hours after your activity ends. End result: better blood sugar control. In one amazing 2012 study from Maastricht University in the Netherlands, published in the journal *Diabetes Care,* people with diabetes who exercised at a moderate pace for a half-hour just 3 or 4 days a week slashed their exposure to the damaging effects of high blood sugar.[3] The researchers found that while nonexercisers' blood sugar levels spiked to high levels nearly 8 hours each day, exercisers' blood sugar levels stayed in a healthy range almost 3 hours longer every day—a difference that lowered their long-term risk for diabetes-related complications like nerve damage, vision loss, and kidney problems.

> The benefits of exercise can last for hours after your activity ends. End result: better blood sugar control.

Reduce insulin resistance. Exercise makes your cells more likely to obey insulin's "Hey, open up and let the blood sugar in!" messages more readily. This benefit kicks in after just a week of exercise. Insulin resistance fell by 30 percent in one 2007 Tufts University study.[4]

Drop cortisol levels. Remember what we said about this stress hormone in Chapter 1: High levels of it flame inflammation and worsen blood sugar control. Exercise helps reduce the emotional stress that can lead to these chronically high cortisol levels. Almost any form of exercise or physical activity can be a natural stress-buster.

Build calorie-hungry muscle. Muscle burns calories around the clock. It draws sugar and fatty acids from your bloodstream, burning them for energy. There's some disagreement over exactly how many calories each pound of muscle burns, with some people saying only about 5 calories a day and others saying it's closer to 50 calories. Either way, that's much more than your fat stores, which burn few calories at all.

Trouble is, we start losing some of our muscle mass

every decade beginning in our mid-thirties. With less muscle on board to burn calories, losing weight and keeping it off can be more difficult. This is why building muscle with strength training is so important.

Melt more belly fat. In a 2006 Johns Hopkins University study, 104 women and men who walked on a treadmill or rode exercise bikes 3 days a week and did a strength-training routine lost 18 percent of their belly fat.[5] This combination beats walking alone. In a 2010 study published in the *International Journal of Sport Nutrition and Exercise Metabolism,* women who walked and performed a simple strength-training routine 3 days a week slimmed their midsections 2 percent more than those who just walked.

Improve heart health. Your heart and arteries age faster if you have blood sugar problems, thanks to high blood pressure, high cholesterol, inflammation, stiff arteries, and other effects, say University of Colorado experts. In a 2011 review, these experts noted that cardiovascular health declines twice as fast in people with diabetes as in people without diabetes. The antidote? Aerobic exercise plus strength training, which the researchers say may slow the damage.[6]

Need less medication for high cholesterol and high blood pressure. That's important because, as we've mentioned, some of these meds can cause weight gain. In a 2012 National Institutes of Health study of 5,145 people with diabetes, those who followed a healthy diet and got regular exercise lost weight and needed less medication—and less expensive, name-brand medication—for optimal control of their cholesterol and blood pressure levels.[7]

Improve total body health. Exercise can strengthen your bones, lower risk for certain cancers, improve your sleep, and lift your mood.

FAQ: WHAT ABOUT EXERCISING WITH DIABETES? SHOULD I EAT BEFOREHAND?

Before exercising, you should always take your blood sugar readings, especially if you are taking any medication to lower your blood sugar. If your blood sugar is 100 mg/dl or less (or if you are prone to hypoglycemia) and you will be exercising intensely for 30 minutes or longer, you should plan a carbohydrate-containing snack or meal before your workout (a fruit, starch, dairy item, or even a vegetable). Test your blood sugar directly before exercise, at the completion of exercise, and an hour after exercise if you tend to experience post-exercise hypoglycemia.

The Elements of the 2 Day Diabetes Exercise Program

Not yet active? Goose bump-raising flashbacks of sixth-grade dodgeball still haunting your dreams? Not to worry. We promise to start you slowly (and get that icky image out of your head!). This program is a mix of aerobic exercise and strength training—an unbeatable combo scientists worldwide have identified as the perfect recipe for improved health and vitality. No humiliation required. As always, though, we do suggest that you check with your doctor before beginning any new plan.

Our exercise program includes three important components:

1. **Walking** to burn calories, lift mood, and encourage your muscles to pull sugar out of your bloodstream and burn it for energy. The prescription: 30 to 45 minutes, 3 to 5 days a week.

2. **Strength training** to build muscle. When you have more muscle on board, you'll mop up more blood sugar with every step you take and every move you make all day long. This will improve your insulin sensitivity and help you better manage blood sugar. It will also help you burn more calories 24/7. The prescription: 20 minutes, two times a week.

3. **A belly-burning routine.** You'll do it in conjunction with your strength-training program to flatten your midsection. This routine will help you target everyone's number one trouble spot, and it will also allow you to target that deep belly fat that tends to raise levels of inflammation. The prescription: two times a week, with your strength-training routine.

FAQ: SHOULD I DRINK EXTRA WATER BEFORE, DURING, AND/OR AFTER I EXERCISE?

Since you lose water through sweating when exercising, it's important to replace this water loss to stay hydrated. For every 30 minutes of exercise, you should drink an additional 8 ounces of water (and for very intense exercise or on very hot days, you should drink an extra 8 ounces for every 15 minutes of exercise).

✳ What Our Test Panelists Are Saying about Exercise

Use the following tips and inspiration from our test panelists to fuel your success.

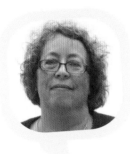

"When I went to my doctor to talk about menopause, she said I needed to exercise for an hour and a half a day—now, don't you just want to just give up in that moment? I mean, really. But this plan is working. My weight is dropping. My blood sugar is dropping. And I'm living on it. I feel like I can do it forever."

—**Karen Lerch**

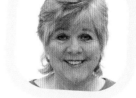

"Getting your family to join you in the diet and the exercise really helps. My kids and I are all going to run or walk a 5-K coming up. It's great to have a goal—and people to share it with."

—**Dianne Barnum**

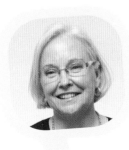

"I figured that my engines would be burning a lot slower the day after depriving my body of fuel on a Power Burn Day. Instead, I woke up early those mornings like I had been shot from a gun. On Tuesdays, that meant I got into the gym early and got in a good workout on the elliptical."

—**Jeanne Plekon**

The 2 Day Diabetes Diet Walking Plan

Aerobic exercise is any activity that requires the use of large muscles and makes your heart beat faster. Walking briskly, hiking, running, climbing stairs, swimming, doing water aerobics, bicycling, ice or inline skating, playing basketball or volleyball or other sports, cross-country skiing—all are aerobic exercise. If you have a favorite on the list, by all means keep doing it. If you don't, walking regularly is the easiest, least expensive way to start a weekly routine that includes aerobic exercise.

Your goal is to walk 30 to 45 minutes a day, 3 to 5 days a week. But you don't have to begin there. Here's a sample schedule that starts with 10 minutes of walking and builds you up to 45 minutes over a period of 6 weeks.

WEEK	WALKING TIME
1	10 minutes, 3 days a week
2	20 minutes, 3 days a week
3	30 minutes, 3 days a week
4	40 minutes, 3 days a week
5	45 minutes, 3 days a week
6	45 minutes, 3 to 5 days a week

Studies have shown that you don't have to walk for 30 to 45 minutes at a time to reap the benefits—only that your total walking time per day should add up to that amount. What that means is that, if you find it tough to squeeze a 30-minute walk into your schedule, don't sweat it. Simply walk for 10 minutes at lunch and 20 minutes after work. Or, walk for 10 minutes after every meal. The total time counts, not the duration of every walk.

Stretch regularly to increase the flow of blood and oxygen to your muscles, improve your flexibility, reduce any soreness associated with your power walks, and speed your recovery. And why wouldn't you? It just feels delicious. These four poses were chosen because they target the large muscles of the lower body most used by walkers. Try them after a particularly intense walk. Ahhh. . . .

Post-Walk Stretches

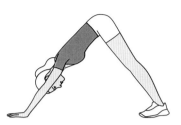

DOWNWARD-FACING DOG POSE

This classic stretches your Achilles tendons, calves, hamstrings, back, shoulders, and arms.

1 Inhale, and place your hands and knees on a mat with your fingers spread wide and your hands shoulder-width apart. As you exhale, lift your knees off the floor, sending your hips towards the ceiling.

2 Press your palms down and back and stretch through your shoulders, drawing your navel into your spine. Stretch through your heels. Hold for three to five breaths.

Note: For tight hamstrings, bend at your knees, and press your torso towards your thighs.

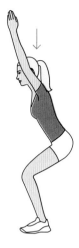

CHAIR POSE

Walkers tend to have tight outer quad muscles, which this pose targets.

1 Stand with your back straight and your big toes touching. Roll your shoulders back, inhale, and reach your arms over your head, keeping your shoulders rolled back.

2 Exhale, bend your knees, and sit your tailbone back as if you were planning to sit down on a chair. Concentrate on drawing your navel to your spine. Hold for three to five breaths, staying in the position longer as your strength and stamina improve.

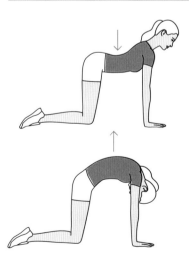

CAT-CAMEL POSE

This one stretches your hips, hamstrings, and lower back.

1 Get down on your hands and knees on a mat with your palms flat on the floor and shoulder-width apart. Relax your core so that your lower back and abdomen are in their natural positions.

2 Gently arch your lower back, then lower your head between your shoulders and raise your upper back toward the ceiling, rounding your spine. Hold for three breaths. Move back and forth slowly, without pushing at either end of the movement.

Post-Walk Stretches continued

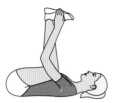

HAPPY BABY POSE
If you have tight hips and a tight lower back like most walkers do, this relaxing pose should make you happy.

1 Begin by lying flat on your back on a mat. Bend both your knees, and grasp the edges of your flexed feet in both hands, keeping your arms to the outside of your legs.

2 Gently use your upper body to press both knees to the floor just below your armpits. Try not to tense your shoulders or chest. Just keep everything relaxed. Hold for five breaths. To release, let go of your feet, and straighten your legs to the floor.

The 2 Day Diabetes Diet Strength-Training Moves

Along with walking, we want you to try some easy strength-training exercises—most don't even require weights! You'll simply use the resistance of your own body to help tone and strengthen your muscles. Make sure you are doing these exercises only on Nourishment Days, especially in the beginning of the diet.

This set of nine exercises couldn't be simpler. All you need is a pair of sneakers, comfortable clothing, and a few everyday objects—a towel or exercise mat for exercises done while sitting or lying on the floor; a chair, table, or countertop for support for a few moves; and the stairs in your home. Some exercises incorporate a light dumbbell, but you won't need one to begin with. They take 20 minutes, tops. And since you can do these exercises anywhere—in a hotel room while you're traveling, behind your office door at work, or in your living room, bedroom, or den—you'll have no excuse not to fit them into your day.

The timing. We've broken the workout into three sequences, which take about 5 to 7 minutes each, so that in the beginning weeks, you can do just one sequence on a particular day. You might do the Upper-

Body Sequence on Monday, the Core Sequence on Wednesday, and the Lower-Body Sequence on Saturday, for instance. The three moves in each sequence don't even have to be done at the same time. You could spend just a couple of minutes doing one move in the morning, then spend a few more minutes doing the other two moves in the evening. As you get stronger, start doing the whole routine at once, and do it twice a week.

The rules. Perform 8 to 12 repetitions of each exercise, then rest for 30 to 60 seconds in between exercises. Once the moves become easy, you can add a second set of repetitions. You'll also find tips for taking many of these moves up a notch once you get strong enough that even two sets of repetitions are easy.

One suggestion. Don't repeat the same exercise 2 days in a row. Muscles need time to rest and repair themselves between strength-training sessions. You'll get better results if you give each muscle group a day or two off before working it again.

Upper-Body Sequence

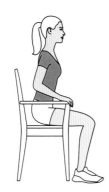 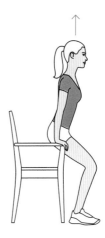

ARMCHAIR DIP

① Sit in a sturdy armchair with your back straight and your feet flat on the floor about hip-width apart. Place your hands on the chair's arms about even with the front of your body.

② Using mostly your arms but assisting with your legs, push yourself out of the chair to a full standing position, letting go of the chair as you stand.

③ Lower yourself back into the chair, grasping the arms of the chair with your hands as you slowly come down, using your arm muscles to return to the starting position.

Note: For a variation, maintain your hold on the arms of the chair until your arms are fully extended, then slowly lower yourself back into the chair.

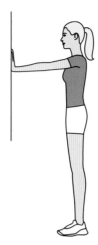 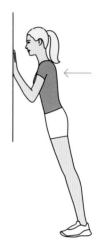

WALL PUSH-UP

1 Stand with your feet shoulder-width apart about 12 to 18 inches from a wall. Place your hands on the wall about shoulder-width apart at chest level, with your palms flat and your fingers pointed toward the ceiling.

2 Slowly lower your chin toward the wall, allowing your elbows to bend to the side. Pause, then smoothly push back from the wall to the starting position.

Note: As you lower yourself to the wall, keep your elbows out to the side. That works the chest muscles better than keeping your elbows close to the body, which shifts the load more to the triceps muscles of the arms. If you feel pain in your hands or wrists, try placing your hands farther apart or closer together on the wall.

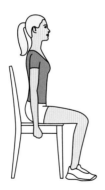 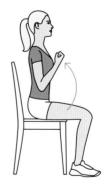

SEATED BICEPS CURL

1 Sit up with your back straight on the front half of an armless chair. Your feet should be flat on the floor and your arms hanging down by your side.

2 Smoothly bend your elbows, keeping them positioned at your side, raising your hands toward your shoulders while rotating your

palms a quarter turn so they face your shoulder at the top of the movement. Smoothly return to the starting position.

Note: If this exercise becomes too easy, try performing it while holding light dumbbells. Start with 1- or 2-pound weights, and gradually increase the weight of the dumbbells as your strength and fitness improve.

Core Sequence

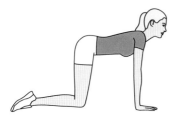
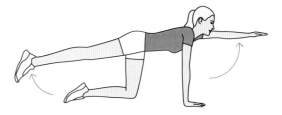

BIRD DOG

1 Get down on your hands and knees on the floor, a rug, or an exercise mat.

2 Extend your right leg out behind you, keeping your foot a few inches off the floor as you straighten your knee.

3 As you're extending your right leg, reach out straight in front of you with your left arm. Return to the starting position and repeat with the other leg and arm to complete one repetition.

4 Continue alternating legs and arms until you finish a set.

Note: Try to keep your back as flat as possible during the movement. If this exercise becomes too easy, try this variation: When you extend your leg behind you, raise it until your leg is parallel to the floor.

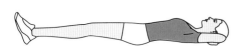
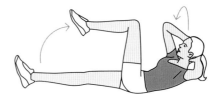

BICYCLE

1 Lie flat on your back with your legs straight and your hands lightly touching your ears behind your head.

2 Lift your head off the floor, and bring your left knee toward your head, stopping when your knee is about waist level and your thigh is perpendicular to the floor. At the same time, bring your right elbow toward the elevated knee so that your torso twists slightly and your elbow and knee are as close as possible over your abdomen.

3 Slowly return to the starting position. Rest for 1 second, and repeat with the opposite limbs.

Note: This exercise should take about 5 seconds, with 2 seconds to bring your knee and elbow close, and 3 seconds to return. As you become stronger, reduce the resting time for a more difficult workout. All motions should be smooth and controlled, which keeps resistance on your muscles and improves your strength and tone more quickly.

Core Sequence continued

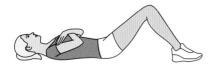 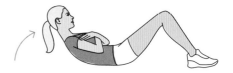

ABDOMINAL CURL

1 Lie on your back with feet flat on the floor, your knees bent, and your arms folded across your chest with each hand touching the opposite shoulder.

2 Raising your head, use your abdominal muscles to pull your shoulders off the floor so you can look at the top of your knees. Keep enough space to fit a baseball between your chin and chest.

3 Slowly lower your shoulders back to the floor.

Lower-Body Sequence

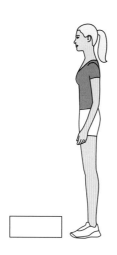 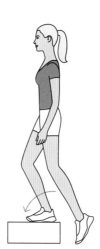 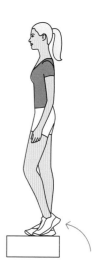

STAIR STEP-UP

1 Stand in front of a step with both feet on the floor about hip-width apart.

2 Place your right foot solidly on the stair, and step up. Bring your left foot up, and touch it lightly on the step before lowering it back to the floor.

3 Step down with your right foot.

4 Step up with your left foot, bringing your right foot up and touching it lightly on the step, then lowering it back to the floor. Alternate steps in this way, counting one repetition when each foot has stepped up one time.

Note: Make this exercise more difficult by using only one foot instead of alternating. For example, use the right foot to step up, step down, then step up again rather than alternating with the left foot. When you've finished a set of step-ups with the right foot, do a set with the left.

Lower-Body Sequence continued

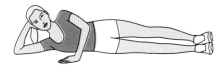

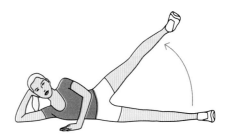

SIDE HIP ABDUCTION

1 Lie on your right side with both legs extended and resting one on top of the other, supporting your head with your right hand.

2 In a smooth and controlled motion, lift your fully extended left leg straight up as high as you comfortably can. Then lower it back to the starting position. After one set, repeat with the other leg.

Note: If you feel unstable in the starting position, try bending your lower leg to provide a wider base of support. If this exercise becomes too easy, try performing it while wearing light ankle weights. Start with half-pound or 1-pound weights, then increase the weight as your strength and fitness improve.

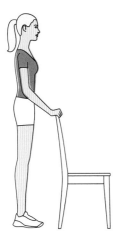

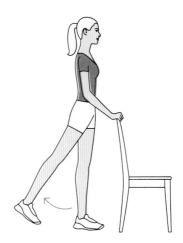

STANDING HIP EXTENSION

1 Stand facing a chair or counter with your feet about hip-width apart, lightly holding on to the chair or counter.

2 Without bending your knee, move your right leg from the hip back behind you. Return slowly to the starting position. After one set, repeat with the other leg.

Note: Don't lock the knee of the leg you're standing on; instead, keep it slightly bent. While the motion is pendulum-like, you shouldn't let momentum do the work. Perform the move slowly, especially during the return phase. If this exercise becomes too easy, try it while wearing a light ankle weight.

The 2 Day Diabetes Diet Belly Burners

These three belly-tightening moves will build your abdominal muscles to shrink your belly and reduce the visceral fat that is so dangerous for people with or at risk for diabetes. Add them twice a week to your strength-training routine. Either include them all at once, or try just one to start, gradually adding another and then another as your strength and fitness improve. You'll have a toned tummy in no time!

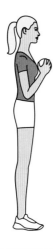

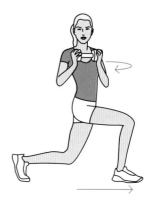

LEG LUNGES WITH ROTATION

1 Stand with your back straight and your feet about hip-width apart, grasping a light dumbbell with both hands. Extend your arms so that you're holding the dumbbell away from your body; keep your elbows straight but not locked. Take a giant step forward with your right foot, and, bracing your abdominal muscles, twist your torso to the right as you bend your right knee at a 90-degree angle. Your right thigh should be parallel to the floor, and your right knee directly over your right foot. Make sure your right knee does not extend beyond your right foot.

2 Twist back to center and push off with your right foot so that you return to the starting position.

3 Repeat, stepping forward with your left leg and twisting toward your left. That's one repetition. Repeat 8 to 12 times.

Note: If this exercise feels too difficult, start by doing it without the dumbbell, simply placing your hands on your hips. As you become accustomed to the movement, add the dumbbell.

Belly Burners continued

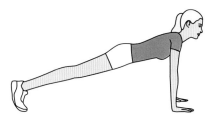

THE PLANK

1 Lie on your belly on the floor, a rug, or an exercise mat like you would if you were getting ready to do a push-up. Press up so that your body is supported by your toes and your hands, keeping them flat on the floor, directly beneath your shoulders. Your body should form a straight line from your head to your feet, without sagging in the middle.

2 Hold for 15 to 30 seconds, then relax.

Note: As your strength and fitness improve, increase the time you hold the Plank from 30 seconds to 1 minute. For even more difficulty, try raising one leg while you hold the Plank. For variety, you can perform planks positioned on your side (the Side Plank) and resting on your forearms (the Elbow Plank). No matter what style of plank you do, your body should always form a straight line from your head to your feet.

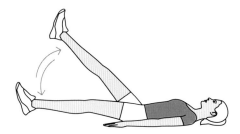

LEG FLUTTERS

1 Lie on your back on the floor, a rug, or an exercise mat with your arms extended at your sides. Keeping your legs straight, raise them so that they form a 45-degree angle with the mat. Flutter your legs by alternately raising them up and down. Do not let your feet touch the floor.

2 Flutter for 30 seconds or do 20 flutters, then relax.

Note: As your strength and fitness improve, extend the time you're fluttering from 30 seconds to 60 seconds; work up to 90 seconds or 45 Leg Flutters. You can also increase the difficulty of the exercise by raising your shoulders off the floor while you flutter.

CHAPTER 12

Find Lasting Success on the 2 Day Diabetes Diet

The key to success on this plan—dieting just 2 days a week—is also the secret to keeping the weight off. Learn how to stay healthy for life!

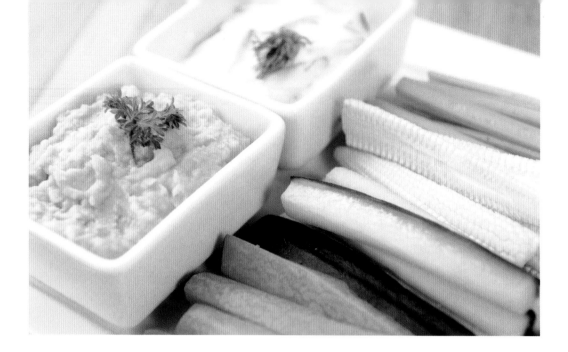

So now you've read through this whole book, and you're familiar with the concepts behind the 2 Day Diabetes Diet. Maybe you've already started the program. Perhaps you've dropped a lot of weight and are nearing your goal. Chances are you're wondering how long you should keep this up as well as how you can make sure this is the last diet you'll ever start. If you've tried other diets in the past, or struggled with managing your diabetes, you may be concerned that the 2 Day Diabetes Diet could become another failed attempt. What does it take to achieve lasting success?

Losing weight and keeping it off is possible. You can succeed with the 2 Day Diabetes Diet. Here's what you need to know.

Counting Down to Your Goal

Keep following any phase of the 2 Day Diabetes Diet as long as needed to reach your goal. That might be just a few weeks if you don't have many pounds to lose, or many, many months if you've got a lot of weight to drop.

Every once in a while, as life intervenes, you can, of course, take a break. Maybe you decide, for instance, not to power burn while on vacation or during a temporarily busy period of life. That's perfectly okay. Just get right back on the plan as soon as you can so you can keep seeing lower numbers on the scale.

We actually recommend that you stay on a version of the 2 Day Diabetes Diet for the rest of your life. After awhile, you'll probably find that sticking to the 2 Day Diabetes Diet becomes second nature. But at the beginning, as you adjust your eating habits to the Power Burn Days/Nourishment Days cycle, you may find yourself wrestling with food cravings or hunger pangs from time to time. Or you might find weight loss hard to start. Maybe you'll hit a plateau or certain life issues will keep you from staying on track. In the following pages, you'll find everything you need to know to solve the top problems you are likely to experience.

Problem #1: I Can't Stop Thinking about Food on Power Burn Days!

Spacing out the Power Burn Days by placing Nourishment Days in between will help. Here are some other suggestions.

Set a timer. Food cravings can feel overwhelming. But they're usually short lived, and if you can buy yourself 20 minutes or so, you'll find they fade away. So when you're gripped by an urge to dive head first into a bag of chips or pump quarters into the vending machine as if you're in Vegas, find a short-term task to keep you busy. Take a walk, write some e-mails, call a friend, work on a hobby. You'll probably find that cravings have subsided by the time you're finished.

Keep a craving diary. If food cravings are a recurring problem, try jotting down the time of day they occurred, what you were doing, how long the cravings lasted, and how you handled them. See page 300 for a sample journal page. Over time, you may see patterns that will help you plan. For example, if you find that cravings are worst in late afternoon, you might have your snack then, or keep yourself busy running errands that keep you away from tempting treats.

Give your taste buds a palate cleanser. Brushing your tongue can take your mouth's mind off of the fridge. Indulge yourself and buy several different flavors and kinds of toothpaste—cinnamon, wintergreen, straight-up teeth-whitening. If you're still craving a snack, just tell yourself, "As soon as I brush my teeth, I can head to the kitchen." Chances are, the craving will get washed down the bathroom sink.

Shrink your plates. Believe it or not, studies show that we tend to eat more food when we eat from larger plates and bowls. Larger tableware seems to make the food portions seem smaller, so we end up piling on more food and chowing down without a second thought. But smaller plates make portion sizes seem larger, and you'll actually feel fuller and more satisfied while eating less.

> Take your time to enjoy the flavor of the delicious recipes we've created for you.

Eat slowly and enjoy. The more satisfying your meals, the less likely you are to experience cravings for the rest of the day. There's more to feeling satisfied than having a full stomach. Your body has several mechanisms in place designed to help you stop eating once you've consumed enough food to fuel your cells for a few hours. Nerves near the stomach, for instance, tell the brain "Turn off the appetite" once they stretch to support the weight of a heavier, food-filled stomach. Various hormones—such as insulin—rise as you eat. Others, like ghrelin, fall. All of this tells your brain to turn off that empty feeling in the pit of the stomach.

The problem: There's a bit of lag time. If you wolf down a meal, you may end up gobbling extra calories and reaching for more food before your brain hears "Stop!" Conversely, taking your time as you eat and enjoying every bite will help you to feel full sooner. One study found that eating a meal over the course of 30 minutes led people to report feeling fuller, compared to people who ate the same meal in 5 minutes. Other research shows that people who eat slowly feel full with 10 percent fewer calories. So take your time to enjoy the flavor of the delicious recipes we've created for you (if you don't, you'll hurt our feelings). And avoid watching TV while you eat, or doing other things that will make you rush or distract you from the sensations of eating.

Problem #2: I'm Used to Eating All Night Long. Now I Don't Know What to Do with Myself!

We're not going to lie to you: If you're used to munching until midnight, at the very start of the 2 Day Diabetes Diet, those Power Burn Days can be a bit challenging to manage—especially after your evening meal, when it can seem a long way to breakfast. But going to bed with an empty stomach will allow your body to sink into deep rest, recharge, and rev up for the next day's fat burning. Try some of these tricks to get your mind off of the evening cravings.

Shine your sink. And turn off the kitchen light. As soon as dinner is over, mentally hang the "closed for business" sign up in your kitchen. Hang a small mirror on your cupboard door, so you'll see yourself if you head in for some crackers.

Take a homemade steam bath. When you feel yourself starting to crave a bowl of ice cream, head to the bathroom and crank the hot water instead. Take as hot a shower as you can stand, and then put your pajamas on right away—your bed will draw you in that much faster.

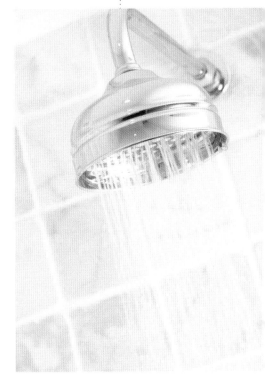

Make a date. Tell your spouse to meet you in the bedroom right after the dinner dishes are done or the kids are asleep, even if it's only 8 p.m.—in fact, especially if it's only 8 p.m. Plenty of time for adult play before lights out!

Or just put yourself to bed. If you're not in the mood for love, still head to the bedroom (i.e., well away from the kitchen). Many a well-intentioned dieter is tripped up by late-night munchies. Cut those cravings off at the knees by setting your bedroom lights on a timer to go off an hour earlier than normal. This not only will keep you out of the kitchen, it will give you some extra shut eye, which is important for keeping hunger and cravings in check 24/7.

Problem #3: The Scale Keeps Giving Me the Same Readout!

There are a few avenues to explore. Have you started the 2 Day Diabetes Diet exercise plan yet? If not, now's a great time to do so. This will keep the pounds peeling off. If you've already added exercise, consider upping the intensity or changing up your routine. The more variety in your exercise routine, the better the boost to your metabolism.

Now's also a great time to start keeping a food journal to make sure you're doing everything right. You're only human. So perhaps you're not hewing as closely to the 2 Day Diabetes Diet plan as you think you are.

You're busy, you're pressed for time, you did miss that one day of exercising, and sometimes you don't test your blood sugar level, and you went off the diet once last week, or was it twice, or three times . . . ?

Recording what you're doing will help you stay accountable.

Anyway, it's not about feeling inadequate because you didn't follow instructions. The point is, when the numbers aren't moving in the right direction, it's a good idea to pay attention to what you're eating, portion sizes, and how the food is prepared—just long enough to be sure that some details aren't slipping through the cracks.

It may seem tedious at first, but writing down what you eat is well worth the time. Recording what you're doing will help you stay accountable, help you stay focused on your goals, and also help you to see how food, sleep, stress, and other issues might be affecting your weight and your blood sugar. We've provided a sample journal page for you on page 292. You can photocopy it if you like or simply use it as a guide and adapt it.

Either way, use these tips for log-keeping success.

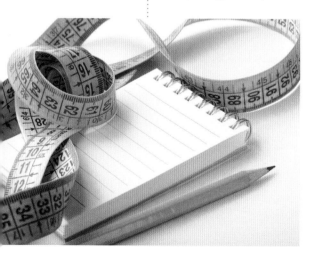

▶ Weigh yourself at least once a week. Try to weigh yourself at the same time and under the same conditions each week (for instance, right after waking up and before having breakfast).

- Note the date, what week and day of the program you are on, and whether you are doing a Power Burn or Nourishment Day.
- When you are recording your foods, write not only what you ate, but also the portion sizes.
- If you choose, you can check off how many servings of each food you have had at each meal and total them at the end of the day. This is especially helpful to keep you on track if you choose to make changes to the meal options or need to eat out.
- In addition to food intake, your fluid intake can also impact your weight and blood sugar levels. Record how much water, tea, juice, or other fluids (aside from the bouillon in your meals) you drink each day.
- Write down any exercise or other physical activity you do and make note of the time of day, duration, and any other details about the exercise you find helpful. You can also list your relaxation exercises here, and when you do them.
- Test your blood sugar regularly to see how food, stress, and other factors affect it—and also how your blood sugar affects your appetite. Consider recording the following if you don't do so already: fasting blood sugar (test immediately upon waking up); pre-meal blood sugar (test right before eating a meal); and post-meal blood sugar (test 2 hours after a meal, counting 2 hours from the time of your first bite).
- Finally, record any additional notes or questions that you think might help you later on. Are you experiencing hunger/ cravings? Have you had any symptoms of hypoglycemia? Do you have more energy before or after exercising? Do you find the relaxation exercises helpful?

WHAT'S YOUR PERFECT WEIGHT?

The number you want to see on the scale and the number you can maintain without starving yourself might be two different numbers. Many of us start a weight loss plan with a predetermined number in mind, and often that number is unrealistic—perhaps it's based on your high school weight, or a celebrity's report weight. While may be possible to shrink your body down to that predetermined weight, you might find that it requires you to eat such small portions that you decide that it's just not worth it.

Remember, it only takes a small amount of weight loss to dramatically lower blood sugar and improve health. If the scale is stuck and you've already tried everything to get it moving, ask yourself, "Have I reached my goal?" It's quite possible that you have, and that means it's time to celebrate!

2 Day Diabetes Diet Daily Food Log and Activity Journal

Name _____ Weight _____

Date _____ Week _____ Day _____ Power Burn ☐ or Nourishment ☐

Time	Food Eaten	Veg	Fruit	Starch	Protein	Fat	Dairy	Bouillon	Treats
Totals:									

Fluids: _____

TIME	EXERCISE OR ACTIVITY	DURATION/ REPS

	TIME	BLOOD SUGAR
Fasting (test on-waking up)		
Pre-meal (test right before eating meal)		
Post-meal (test 2 hours after meal)		

Additional Notes/Comments: _____

_____

Problem #4: The Scale Is *Still* Giving Me the Same Readout!

So you kept the food log and now you know: You are eating according to plan. But your log might hint that other issues might be amiss. Using your log as a guide, consider whether any of the following problems are hindering your success.

Your medications. New medications and changes in medication dosages can impact weight. For instance, someone whose blood sugar was running around 300mg/dl (16.7 mmol/l), starts on meds, and brings the blood sugar down to 150mg/dl (8.3 mmol/l) in a short period of time may see no weight loss or even a slight gain as the excess sugar in the bloodstream enters the cells and is metabolized. So if you've changed medication or recently had a notable change in blood sugar levels, you may need to spend a few weeks in your new situation before the 2 Day Diabetes Diet produces results. Touch base with your doctor or certified diabetes educator. (And of course, if you've had a large change in blood sugar levels that you can't explain, definitely talk to your physician about it.)

It's also possible that medication you take for your diabetes is sabotaging your weight loss. Insulin, for example, can increase appetite and store fat. If you suspect that's the case, don't just stop taking your medicine, and don't experiment with changing the dose. Talk to your doctor first. If there's not an alternate medication you can take, odds are the 2 Day Diabetes Diet will still work. You'll just need to be extra careful about sticking to the meal plan and tracking your progress and be patient. It may take longer to reach your goal weight, but you will get there if you follow the plan diligently.

Your sleep hygiene (or lack of it). If you don't always get as much sleep as you need, you're not the only one. In polls, 30 to 40 percent of adults say they have some symptoms of insomnia, and about 10 to 15 percent of adults say they have chronic insomnia.

And if you've ever noticed that you feel hungrier on days when you're particularly tired, you're not imagining things either. There's evidence that lack of sleep affects the levels of ghrelin, the hunger hormone we mentioned in Chapter 1. It causes ghrelin to stay elevated, making you feel hungry long after you should feel full. Do the following:

- **Get a sleep test.** People who are overweight can suffer from a condition called sleep apnea, a sleep-related breathing disorder that leads individuals to repeatedly stop breathing for short periods during sleep. Those pauses in breathing, which can last for 10 seconds at a time, disrupt sleep and leave you tired the next day. Talk to your physician about options for diagnosing and treating the problem.

- **Cut back on caffeine.** Too much caffeine during the day can make it harder to fall asleep at night, which makes you all the more tired the next day, which makes you seek out more caffeine . . . you get the idea. Add all of this to the effects of sleep on appetite, and you can see why a good night's sleep may be as important for weight loss as a healthy diet and regular exercise.

- **Be consistent with your sleep and wake times.** The closer you stick to the same bedtime and wakeup schedule—even on weekends—the more likely your body will switch from wake to sleep when the time comes. If you take a nap during the day, limit it to 30 to 45 minutes.

- **Use the bed for bed stuff only.** Don't be one of those people who watches TV, eats snacks, does paperwork, makes phone calls, and does a half-dozen other things while reclining in bed. Your body needs to reflexively associate your bed with sleep, so reserve the bed for sleeping, sex, and light reading before dozing off. Everything else should take place elsewhere, preferably in a different room.

- **Decompress and descreen before sleep.** Just like your car, your body doesn't like to shift from fifth gear to park in a split second. So build some time into your evening schedule—maybe an hour or more—to stop working, turn down the lights, slow down the conversation, and generally signal to your psyche that the day is winding down. Avoid anything that stresses or stimulates you, and turn off all screens: TV, computer, tablet, cell phone, everything! Not only do these things tend to stimulate, there's evidence that bathing your eyes in the light from electronic devices makes it harder to relax. Instead, listen to some soothing music or do some pleasant reading (but not on an electronic, backlit device).

- **Create quiet.** Sometimes we get so used to the things in our environment that we no longer notice them, at least consciously. But that doesn't mean they don't affect us. Familiar noises that you don't think much about, like traffic sounds or a dripping faucet, could be stealing your sleep. If you can't eliminate distracting noises, make your room quieter by closing windows, eliminating noisy appliances, or using earplugs or a white-noise device (or run a fan or air conditioner to mask sounds).

- **Balance light and darkness.** Your sleep clock is strongly affected by how much light you're exposed to during the day. Try to spend some time outdoors every day if possible, so your body clock gets a good dose of natural light. If that's not possible, a light box or similar device that produces illumination similar to sunlight can help keep your biological clock on schedule. At night, make your bedroom as dark as possible. Avoid bright light if you wake up in the middle of the night; use a night-light if you need to get out of bed.

- **Warm up to cool down.** A warm bath is not only relaxing, it triggers a temperature drop afterwards that can signal your body to sleep. Try making it part of your pre-bedtime routine.

- **Keep a cool bedroom.** Most people sleep better in a room that's kept slightly cool, so experiment with turning down the thermostat until you reach the zone that's right for you. Blankets and bedding will help you adjust your warmth level without getting too hot to sleep.

- **Review your mattress.** If it's been a while since you bought your mattress, it may be time for a new one. Shop around; research shows that testing a mattress for at least 15 minutes at the store makes a big difference in finding one that's comfortable. Also try different kinds of pillows and bedding.

> Build some time into your evening to signal your psyche that the day is winding down.

▶ **Avoid eating right before bed, except for a light snack.**
Large meals close to bedtime can make it harder to stay asleep.
Also avoid alcohol, which makes you sleepy at first but disrupts
sleep later on. Caffeine, even earlier in the day, can make sleep
more difficult. And vigorous exercise should be scheduled for
morning or early afternoon.

▶ **Too much stress.** They don't call it "comfort food" for
nothing. We all have days when we feel overwhelmed, fried,
stressed out. And when that happens, it can seem like the
only cure is a bag of chips or a bowl of ice cream. If you think
stress is your problem, look no farther than the Tension Tamers
showcased in Chapter 10.

Staying at Your Goal Weight

The end of the 2 Day Diabetes Diet is just the beginning. When you reach
your weight-loss goal, you want to stay there. Here's the good news: According to results from the National Weight Control Registry (NWCR)—a
long-running study of weight loss that contains data on more than 10,000
people who've lost weight and successfully kept it off—almost half of the
successful dieters found it easier to keep the weight off than it was to lose
the weight in the first place.[1] So, contrary to popular opinion, if you've
already reached a healthy weight, it could be that the hard part is already over! Another 33 percent said that the difficulty of losing weight
and keeping it off was about the same. Bottom line: There's a perception
that keeping the pounds off once you've shed them is an uphill battle.
But it isn't necessarily so. Nor should you feel that you'll never stay slim
because it's not "in your genes." Seventy percent of these dieters who kept
the weight off had been obese since childhood, and 73 percent had at least
one overweight parent.

If you haven't already started exercising, now's a great time to start.
And if you are already exercising, it's a great idea to keep it up. One

strategy that almost all successful dieters report is exercise. After losing weight, most of the successful reducers (72 percent) burned at least 1,000 calories a week by exercising. Another study using the NWCR database found that dieters who regained weight reported a notable drop in physical activity, burning 800 fewer calories per week over the course of a year. These statistics, and other research, make it clear: To lose weight and keep it off, regular exercise needs to be part of the picture.

In addition to starting an exercise plan, you'll want to make a few small tweaks to your 2 Day Diabetes Diet plan. Do the following:

Drop the Power Burn Days. Continue to follow the 1,500-calorie Nourishment Days diet as a maintenance program for as long as you like. This is a healthy way of eating, not a crash diet. We recommend you continue to have Nourishment Days for the rest of your life. You can keep using the recipes and tips in this book to stay on a healthy track.

Get on the scale at least once a week. This will help you to catch weight gain before it gets out of control. The experts call this "self-monitoring." Most successful reducers check their weight multiple times a week, many every day. Which only makes sense: If your weight is trending upwards, it's easier to make course corrections—exercise more, be stricter about what you eat—if you catch it early. Set a 5-pound weight range to stay within. Everyone's weight fluctuates some, but you don't want your weight to fluctuate more than 5 pounds.

Use Power Burn Days to power down. If you creep above this range, go back to incorporating Power Burn Days again until you are back at your goal.

You worked hard to get here. Remember that every day. It was your hard work and perseverance that allowed you to stick to the plan, overcome barriers, and ultimately conquer blood sugar issues and the excess pounds. Feel good about all you've done.

We're so happy for you. Here's to your dieting success!

2 Day Diabetes Diet Recommended Brands

When you're following a new meal plan, grocery shopping can feel a bit overwhelming. To help you stay on track, here's a list of foods and brands that fit into your 2 Day Diabetes Diet plan. This isn't a complete list, and other brand-name foods that fit your meal plan guidelines can be substituted, as long as they're similar.

Milk/Yogurt

Almond Breeze, original

EdenSoy, original or unsweetened

Silk Pure Almond® Original almond milk

Silk Soymilk, original or vanilla

Soy Dream, original, enriched original, enriched vanilla

2% Chobani Greek yogurt, plain

Dannon, plain all-natural yogurt

Liberté, plain organic 2.5% yogurt

Silk Live! plain soy yogurt

Breads/Buns

Arnold's Sandwich Thins

Food for Life 7 Sprouted Grains English Muffin

Food for Life Ezekiel 4:9 Sprouted Grain Bread

Nature's Own Premium Specialty 100% Whole Grain Bread

Nature's Own 100% Whole Wheat Hot Dog Rolls

Pepperidge Farm 100% Whole Wheat Hoagie Rolls

Pepperidge Farm Deli Flats® 100% Whole Wheat Thin Rolls

Pepperidge Farm Light Style Seven Grain Bread

Thomas Hearty Grains 100% Whole Wheat bagels and English muffins

Vitalicious VitaBuns

Cereals

All-Bran

Cheerios (Original)

Fiber One 80 Calories

Fiber One Original Cereal

Kashi GoLean Crunch! Cereal

McCann's Steel Cut Irish Oatmeal

Total cereal

Crackers

Kashi crackers

Triscuits

Wasa crackers

Pasta/Grains

Annie Chun's Brown Rice Noodles

Bionaturae 100% Stone Ground Whole Durum Wheat Organic Pasta

Bob's Red Mill Organic Whole Grain Quinoa

Hodgson Mill Whole Wheat Couscous

King Arthur Organic 100% Whole Grain Flour

Ronzoni Healthy Harvest Whole Wheat Blend Pasta

Uncle Ben's Natural Whole Grain Brown Rice

Tortillas

Flatout breads (varieties with 90 to 110 calories per serving)

La Tortilla Factory 100 Calorie Whole Wheat Tortilla

Condiments

365 Organic Unsweetened Peanut Butter from Whole Foods

Cedar's Hummus, all flavors

Kraft Good Seasons Italian Vinaigrette with Extra Virgin Olive Oil

Land O'Lakes Butter with Canola Oil

Land O'Lakes Light Butter with Canola Oil

Newman's Own Dressing Lite Red Wine Vinegar & Olive Oil

Newman's Own Olive Oil & Vinegar Dressing

Olivio, light spread

Olivio, original spread

SmartBalance Light Buttery Spread with EVOO

SmartBalance Light Omega-3 Buttery Spread

SmartBalance Light Buttery Spread with Flaxseed Oil

SmartBalance Original Buttery Spread

Smucker's Natural Peanut Butter

Muffins/Waffles

Van's 8 Whole Grains Multigrain waffles

Vitalicious VitaMuffin

Treats

Baked! Ruffles Potato Chips

Bear Naked Granola Cookies, all varieties

Edy's Slow Churned ice cream

Emerald nuts, dry roasted, cocoa roasted, or cinnamon roasted

Glenny's Soy Crisps

Godiva 72% or 85% Cacao Chocolate Bars

Kashi cookies, all varieties

Lindt 70%, 85%, or 90% Cacao Bars

popchips

Sweetriot Dark Chocolate

Sun Chips 6 Grain Medley

Bouillon

Hormel Foods Herb-Ox® bouillon, all varieties

Notes

Introduction

1. R. F. Hamman et al., "Effect of weight loss with lifestyle intervention on risk of diabetes," *Diabetes Care* 29, no. 9 (September 2006): 2102–7.
2. M. Harvie et al., "Intermittent dietary carbohydrate restriction enables weight loss and reduces breast cancer risk biomarkers." Presented at the CTRC-AACR San Antonio Breast Cancer Symposium, December 2011.
3. R. S. Gill et al., "Predictors of attrition in a multidisciplinary adult weight management clinic," *Canadian Journal of Surgery* 55, no. 4 (August 2012): 239–243.
4. K. M. Beavers et al., "Is lost lean mass from intentional weight loss recovered during weight regain in postmenopausal women?" *American Journal of Clinical Nutrition* 93, no. 3 (Sept 2011): 767-774.

Chapter 1

1. M. J. Franz, "The dilemma of weight loss in diabetes," *Diabetes Spectrum* 20, no. 3 (July 2007): 133–36.
2. A. Galassi, K. Reynolds, and J. He, "Metabolic syndrome and risk of cardiovascular disease: A meta-analysis." *American Journal of Medicine* 119, no. 10 (October 2006): 812–19.
3. E. W. Wamsteker et al., "Unrealistic weight-loss goals among obese patients are associated with age and causal attributions," *Journal of the American Dietetic Association* 109, no. 11 (November 2009): 1903–8.
4. See Introduction, note 1.
5. K. M. Flegal, B. I. Graubard, D. F. Williamson, and M. H. Gail, "Excess deaths associated with underweight, overweight, and obesity," *Journal of the American Medical Association* 293, no. 15 (20 April 2005): 1861–67.

Chapter 2

1. P. K. Stein et al., "Caloric restriction may reverse age-related autonomic decline in humans," *Aging Cell* 11, no. 4 (August 2012): 644–50. Epub 2012 May 21.
2. T. E. Meyer et al., "Long-term caloric restriction ameliorates the decline in diastolic function in humans," *Journal of the American College of Cardiology* 47, no. 2 (17 January 2006): 398–402.
3. I. Salim et al., "Impact of religious Ramadan fasting on cardiovascular disease: A systemic review of the literature," *Current Medical Research and Opinion* 29, no. 4 (April 2013): 343–54.
4. M. A. Faris et al., "Intermittent fasting during Ramadan attenuates proinflammatory cytokines and immune cells in healthy subjects," *Nutrition Research* 32, no. 12 (December 2012): 947–55.
5. M. N. Harvie et al., "The effects of intermittent or continuous energy restriction on weight loss and metabolic disease risk markers: A randomised trial in young overweight women." *International Journal of Obesity* 35, no. 5 (May 2011): 714–27.
6. Ibid.

Chapter 3

1. N. Halberg et al., "Effect of intermittent fasting and refeeding on insulin action in healthy men," *Journal of Applied Physiology* 99, no. 6 (December 2005): 2128–36. Epub 2005 July 28.
2. K. A. Varady and M. K. Hellerstein, "Alternate-day fasting and chronic disease prevention: A review of human and animal trials." *American Journal of Clinical Nutrition* 86, no. 1 (July 2007): 7–13.
3. See note 1 above.
4. See Introduction, note 2
5. Ibid.
6. A. Shapiro et al., "Fructose-induced leptin resistance exacerbates weight gain in response to subsequent high fat feeding." *American Journal of Physiology:*

Regulatory, Integrative and Comparative Physiology 295, no. 5 (November 2008): R1370–75. Epub 2008 August 13.

7. L. M. Steffen, D. R. Jacobs Jr., and J. Stevens, "Associations of whole-grain, refined-grain, and fruit and vegetable consumption with risks of all-cause mortality and incident coronary artery disease and ischemic stroke: The Atherosclerosis Risk in Communities (ARIC) Study." *American Journal of Clinical Nutrition* 78, no. 3 (September 2003): 383–90.

8. C. Itsiopoulos, L. Brazionis, and M. Kalmakamis, "Can the Mediterranean diet lower HbA1c in type 2 diabetes? Results from a randomized cross-over study." *Nutrition, Metabolism, and Cardiovascular Diseases* 21, no. 9 (September 2011): 740–47. Epub 2010 July 31.

9. J. Salas-Salvadó, J. Fernández-Ballart, and E. Ros, "Effect of a Mediterranean diet supplemented with nuts on metabolic syndrome status: One-year results of the PREDIMED randomized trial." *Archives of Internal Medicine* 168, no. 22 (8/22 December 2008): 2449–58.

10. K. Esposito, M. I. Maiorino, and M. Ciotola, "Effects of a Mediterranean-style diet on the need for antihyperglycemic drug therapy in patients with newly diagnosed type 2 diabetes: A randomized trial." *Annals of Internal Medicine* 151, no. 5 (1 September 2009): 306–14.

11. D. Schwarzfuchs, R. Golan, and I. Shai, "Four-year follow-up after two-year dietary interventions." *New England Journal of Medicine* 367, no. 14 (4 October 2012): 1373–74.

12. A. E. Field, W. C. Willett, L. Lissner, and G. A. Colditz, "Dietary fat and weight gain among women in the nurses' health study." *Obesity* 15, no. 4 (April 2007): 967–76.

13. P. Schieberle et al., "Identifying substances that regulate satiety in oils and fats and improving low-fat foodstuffs by adding lipid compounds with a high satiety effect; Key findings of the DFG/AiF cluster project; Perception of fat content and regulating satiety: an approach to developing low-fat foodstuffs," 2009–2012.

14. R. Estruch et al., "Primary prevention of cardiovascular disease with a Mediterranean diet." *New England Journal of Medicine* 368, no. 14 (April 4, 2013): 1279-1290.

15. J. M. Fernández-Real et al., "A Mediterranean diet enriched with olive oil is associated with higher serum total osteocalcin levels in elderly men at high cardiovascular risk." *Journal of Clinical Endocrinology and Metabolism* 97, no. 10 (October 2012): 3792-98. Epub 2012 August 1.

16. F. Giugliano et al., "Adherence to Mediterranean diet and erectile dysfunction in men with type 2 diabetes." *Journal of Sexual Medicine* 7, no. 5 (May 2010): 1911–17.

17. F. Giugliano, M. I. Maiorino, and C. Di Palo, "Adherence to Mediterranean diet and sexual function in women with type 2 diabetes." *Journal of Sexual Medicine* 7, no. 5 (May 2010): 1883–90.

18. P. J. Curtis, M. Sampson, and J. Potter, "Chronic ingestion of flavan-3-ols and isoflavones improves insulin sensitivity and lipoprotein status and attenuates estimated 10-year CVD risk in medicated postmenopausal women with type 2 diabetes: A 1-year, double-blind, randomized, controlled trial." *Diabetes Care* 35, no. 2 (February 2012): 226–32.

19. K. Ried et al., "Does chocolate reduce blood pressure? A meta-analysis." *BMC Medicine* 8, no. 39 (28 June 2010).

20. D. Jakubowicz, O. Froy, J. Wainstein, and M. Boaz, "Meal timing and composition influence ghrelin levels, appetite scores and weight loss maintenance in overweight and obese adults." *Steroids* 77, no. 4 (10 March 2012): 323–31.

21. Surwit, R. S., van Tilburg, M. A., Zucker, N., McCaskill, C. C. et al. "Stress management improves long-term glycemic control in type 2 diabetes." *Diabetes Care* 25, no. 1 (January 2002): 30–4.

22. Innes, K. E., Bourguignon, C., Taylor, A. G. "Risk indices associated with the insulin resistance syndrome, cardiovascular disease, and possible protection with yoga: A systematic review." *Journal of the American Board of Family Practice* 18, no. 6 (November–December 2005): 491–519.

23. M. Novak, L. Björck, K. W. Giang, C. Heden-Ståhl, L. Wilhelmsen, A. Rosengren, "Perceived stress and incidence of Type 2 diabetes: a 35-year follow-up study of middle-aged Swedish men," *Diabetic Medicine,* (January 2013); 30 (1): e8-e16.

24. G. Hawley et al., "Sustainability of health and lifestyle improvements following a non-dieting randomised trial in overweight women." *Preventive Medicine* 47, no. 6 (December 2008): 593–99. Epub 2008 September 11.

25. J.-W. van Dijk et al. "Exercise therapy in type 2 diabetes: Is daily exercise required to optimize glycemic control?" *Diabetes Care* 35, no. 5 (May 2012): 948–54. Epub 2012 March 7.

26. K. E. Foster-Schubert, C. M. Alfano, and C. R. Duggan, "Effect of diet and exercise, alone or combined, on weight and body composition in overweight-to-obese postmenopausal women." *Obesity* 20, no. 8 (August 2012): 1628–38. Epub 2011 April 14.

27. K. J. Stewart et al., "Exercise effects on cardiac size and left ventricular diastolic function: Relationships to changes in fitness, fatness, blood pressure and insulin resistance." *Heart* 92, no. 7 (July 2006): 893–98. EPub 2005 November 24.

28. D.-I. Seo et al., "12 weeks of combined exercise is better than aerobic exercise for increasing G\growth hormone in middle-aged women." *International Journal of Sport Nutrition and Exercise Metabolism* 20, no. 1 (February 2010): 21-26.

Chapter 4

1. E. S. Ford and A. H. Mokdad, "Fruit and vegetable consumption and diabetes mellitus incidence among U.S. adults." *Preventive Medicine* 32, no. 1 (January 2001): 33–39.

2. K. Takahashi, C. Kamada, and H. Yoshimura, "Effects of total and green vegetable intakes on glycated hemoglobin A1c and triglycerides in elderly patients with type 2 diabetes mellitus: The Japanese Elderly Intervention Trial." *Geriatrics & Gerontology International* 12, Suppl. 1 (April 2012): 50–58.

3. T. A. Ledoux, M. D. Hingle, and T. Baranowski, "Relationship of fruit and vegetable intake with adiposity: A systematic review." *Obesity Reviews* 12, no. 5 (May 2011): e143–e150. EPub 2010 July 14.

4. J. A. Ello-Martin, L. S. Roe, J. Ledikwe, and A. M. Beach, "Dietary energy density in the treatment of obesity: A year-long trial comparing 2 weight-loss diets." *American Journal of Clinical Nutrition* 85, no. 6 (June 2007): 1465–77.

5. H. C. Hung et al., "Fruit and vegetable intake and risk of major chronic disease." *Journal of the National Cancer Institute* 96, no. 21 (3 November 2004): 1577–84.

6. B. Cevallos-Casals, D. Byrne, W Okie, L. Cisneros-Zevallos, "Selecting new peach and plum genotypes rich in phenolic compounds and enhanced functional properties," *Food Chemistry* 96 (2006): 273-280.

7. R. M. van Dam, N. Naidoo, and R. Landberg, "Dietary flavonoids and the development of type 2 diabetes and cardiovascular diseases: Review of recent findings." *Current Opinion in Lipidology* 24, no. 1 (February 2013): 25–33.

8. N. M. Wedick, A. Pan, and A. Cassidy, "Dietary flavonoid intakes and risk of type 2 diabetes in US men and women." *American Journal of Clinical Nutrition* 95, no. 4 (April 2012): 925–33.

9. K. E. Schroder, "Effects of fruit consumption on body mass index and weight loss in a sample of overweight and obese dieters enrolled in a weight-loss intervention trial." *Nutrition* 26, no. 7–8 (July–August 2010): 727–34. Epub 2009 December 22.

10. S. Alinia, O. Hels, and I. Tetens, "The potential association between fruit intake and body weight—a review." *Obesity Reviews* 10, no. 6 (November 2009): 639–47. Epub 2009 April 1.

11. A. Le Port, A. Gueguen, and E. Kesse-Guyot, "Association between dietary patterns and depressive symptoms over time: A 10-year follow-up study of the GAZEL cohort." *PLoS One* 7, no. 12 (2012): e51593. Epub 2012 December 12.

12. A. J. Sommerfeld, A. L. McFarland, T. M. Waliczek, and J. M. Zajicek, "Growing minds: Evaluating the relationship between gardening and fruit and vegetable consumption in older adults." *HortTechnology* 20, no. 4 (August 2010): 711–17.

13. R. Krikorian et al., "Blueberry supplementation improves memory in older adults." *Journal of Agricultural and Food Chemistry* 58, no. 7 (14 April 2010): 3996–4000.

14. A. S. Lihn, S. B. Pedersen, and B. Richelsen, "Adiponectin: Action, regulation and association to insulin sensitivity." *Obesity Reviews* 6, no. 1 (February 2005): 13–21.

15. T. Wirström et al., "Consumption of whole grain reduces risk of deteriorating glucose tolerance, including progression to prediabetes." *American Journal of Clinical Nutrition* (January 2013): 179–87.

16. A. D. Liese, A. K. Roach, K. C. Sparks, and L. Marquart, "Whole-grain intake and insulin sensitivity: The Insulin Resistance Atherosclerosis Study." *American Journal of Clinical Nutrition* 78, no. 5 (November 2003): 965–71.

17. H. I. Katcher, R. S. Legro, and A. R. Kunselman, "The effects of a whole grain-enriched hypocaloric diet on cardiovascular disease risk factors in men and women with metabolic syndrome." *American Journal of Clinical Nutrition* 87, no. 1 (January 2008): 79–90.

18. Ibid.

19. S. Liu et al., "Whole-grain consumption and risk of coronary heart disease: Results from the Nurses' Health Study." *American Journal of Clinical Nutrition* 70, no. 3 (September 1999): 412–19.

20. K. E. Andersson and P. Hellstrand, "Dietary oats and modulation of atherogenic pathways." *Molecular Nutrition & Food Research* 56, no. 7 (July 2012): 1003–13. Epub 2012 June 12.

21. L. C. Plantinga, D. C. Crews, and J. Coresh, "Prevalence of chronic kidney disease in US adults with undiagnosed diabetes or prediabetes." *Clinical Journal of the American Society of Nephrology* 5, no. 4 (April 2010): 673–82.

22. P. L. Lutsey, L. M. Steffen, and J. Stevens, "Dietary intake and the development of the metabolic syndrome: The Atherosclerosis Risk in Communities study." *Circulation* 117, no. 6 (12 February 2008): 754–61. Epub 2008 January 22.

23. Lutsey, Steffen, and Stevens, "Reduction in the incidence of type 2 diabetes with lifestyle intervention or metformin." *New England Journal of Medicine* 346 (7 February 2002): 393–403.

24. J. Xu et al., "Macronutrient intake and glycemic control in a population-based sample of American Indians with diabetes: The Strong Heart Study." *American Journal of Clinical Nutrition* 86, no. 2 (August 2007): 480–87.

25. A. R. Josse, S. A. Atkinson, M. A. Tarnopolsky, and S. M. Phillips, "Increased consumption of dairy foods and protein during diet- and exercise-induced weight loss promotes fat mass loss and lean mass gain in overweight and obese premenopausal women." *Journal of Nutrition* 141, no. 9 (1 September 2011): 1626–34.

26. T. L. Halton and F. B. Hu, "The effects of high protein diets on thermogenesis, satiety and weight loss: A critical review." *Journal of the American College of Nutrition* 23, no. 5 (October 2004): 373–85.

27. F. Nahab et al., "Racial and geographic differences in fish consumption: The REGARDS Study." *Neurology* 76, no. 2 (11 January 2011): 154–58. Epub 2010 December 22.

28. B. Vessby, M. Uusitupa, and K. Hermansen, "Substituting dietary saturated fat for monounsaturated fat impairs insulin sensitivity in healthy men and women: The KANWU Study." *Diabetologia* 44, no. 3 (March 2001): 312–19.

29. J. A. Paniagua et al., "A MUFA-rich diet improves posprandial glucose, lipid and GLP-1 responses in insulin-resistant subjects." *Journal of the American College of Nutrition* 26, no. 5 (October 2007): 434–44.

30. J. A. Jenkins et al., "Nuts as a replacement for carbohydrates in the diabetic diet." *Diabetes Care* 34, no. 8 (August 2011): 1706–11. Epub 2011 June 29.

31. J. A. Paniagua, A. Gallego de la Sacristana, and I. Romero, "Monounsaturated fat-rich diet prevents central body fat distribution and decreases postprandial adiponectin expression induced by a carbohydrate-rich diet in insulin-resistant subjects." *Diabetes Care* 30, no. 7 (July 2007): 1717–23. Epub 2007 March 23.

32. K. McManus, L. Antinoro, and F. Sacks, "A randomized controlled trial of a moderate-fat, low-energy diet compared with a low-fat, low-energy diet for weight loss in overweight adults." *International Journal of Obesity and Related Metabolic Disorders* 25, no. 10 (October 2001): 1053–11.

33. J. Salas-Salvadó, M. Bulló, and N. Babio, "Reduction in the incidence of type 2 diabetes with the Mediterranean diet: Results of the PREDIMED-Reus nutrition intervention randomized trial." *Diabetes Care* 34, no. 1 (January 2011): 14–19. Epub 2010 October 7.

34. See Chapter 3, note 13.
35. C. M. Benbrook, "Impacts of genetically engineered crops on pesticide use in the U.S.—the first sixteen years." *Environmental Sciences Europe* 24 (28 September 2012).
36. S. Holmberg and A. Thelin, "High dairy fat intake related to less central obesity: A male cohort study with 12 years' follow-up." *Scandinavian Journal of Primary Health Care* (15 January 2013).
37. D. Mozaffarian, H. Cao, and I. B. King, "Trans-palmitoleic acid, metabolic risk factors, and new-onset diabetes in U.S. adults: A cohort study." *Annals of Internal Medicine* 153, no. 12 (21 December 2010).
38. M. A., Pereira, D. R. Jacobs, L. Van Horn, and M. L. Slattery, "Dairy consumption, obesity, and the insulin resistance syndrome in young adults: The CARDIA study." *Journal of the American Medical Association* 287, no. 16 (24 April 2002): 2081–89.
39. F. Fumeron, A. Lamri, and C. Abi Khalil, "Dairy consumption and the incidence of hyperglycemia and the metabolic syndrome: Results from a French prospective study, data from the Epidemiological Study on the Insulin Resistance Syndrome (DESIR)." *Diabetes Care* 34, no. 4 (April 2011): 813–17.
40. A. S. Abargouei, M. Janghorbani, M. Salehi-Marzijarani, and A. Esmaillzadeh, "Effect of dairy consumption on weight and body composition in adults: A systematic review and meta-analysis of randomized controlled clinical trials." *International Journal of Obesity* 36, no. 12 (December 2012): 1485–93.
41. Ibid.
42. R. Roussel et al., "Low water intake and risk for new-onset hyperglycemia." *Diabetes Care* 34, no. 12 (December 2011): 2551–54.
43. B. J. Rolls, L. S. Roe, A. M. Beach, and P. M. Kris-Etherton, "Provision of foods differing in energy density affects long-term weight loss." *Obesity Research* 13, no. 6 (June 2005): 1052–60.
44. R. M. van Dam, W. J. Pasman, and P. Verhoef, "Effects of coffee consumption on fasting blood glucose and insulin concentrations: Randomized controlled trials in healthy volunteers." *Diabetes Care* 27, no. 12 (December 2004): 2990–92.
45. C. Herder, "The InterAct Consortium (2012) tea consumption and incidence of type 2 diabetes in Europe: The EPIC-InterAct case-cohort study." *PLoS ONE* 7, no. 5 (30 May 2012): e36910.
46. J. A. Nettleton et al., "Diet soda intake and risk of incident metabolic syndrome and type 2 diabetes in the Multi-Ethnic Study of Atherosclerosis (MESA)." *Diabetes Care* 32, no. 4 (April 2009): 688–94. Epub 2009 January 16.
47. K. J. Duffey, L. M. Steffen, and L. Van Horn, "Dietary patterns matter: Diet beverages and cardiometabolic risks in the longitudinal Coronary Artery Risk Development in Young Adults (CARDIA) study." *American Journal of Clinical Nutrition* 95, no. 4 (April 2012): 909–15.

Chapter 5

1. S. A. Bajorek and C. M. Morello, "Effects of dietary fiber and low glycemic index diet on glucose control in subjects with type 2 diabetes mellitus." *Annals of Pharmacotherapy* 44, no. 11 (November 2010): 1786–92. Epub 2010 October 19.
2. Ibid.

Chapter 6

1. D. J. A. Jenkins, C. W. C. Kendall, and L.S. A. Augustin, "Effect of legumes as part of a low glycemic index diet on glycemic control and cardiovascular risk factors in type 2 diabetes mellitus: A randomized controlled trial." *Archives of Internal Medicine* 172, no. 21 (26 November 2012): 1653–60.
2. N. Suksomboon, N. Poolsup, S. Boonkaew, and C. C. Suthisisang, "Meta-analysis of the effect of herbal supplement on glycemic control in type 2 diabetes." *Journal of Ethnopharmacology* 137, no. 3 (11 October 2011): 1328–33. Epub 2011 August 5.
3. A. C. Bovell-Benjamin, "Sweet potato: A review of its past, present, and future role in human nutrition." *Advances in Food and Nutrition Research* 52 (2007): 1–59.

4. G. M. Turner-McGrievy and D. Tate, "Weight loss social support in 140 characters or less: use of an online social network in a remotely delivered weight loss intervention," *Translational Behavioral Medicine* Epub January 2013.

Chapter 7

1. J. A. Joseph, B. Shukitt-Hale, and L. M. Willis, "Grape juice, berries, and walnuts affect brain aging and behavior." *Journal of Nutrition* 139, no. 9 (September 2009): 1813S–17S. Epub 2009 July 29.
2. B. W. Bolling, C. Y. Chen, D. L. McKay, and J. B. Blumberg, "Tree nut phytochemicals: Composition, antioxidant capacity, bioactivity, impact factors. A systematic review of almonds, Brazils, cashews, hazelnuts, macadamias, pecans, pine nuts, pistachios and walnuts." *Nutrition Research Reviews* 24, no. 2 (December 2011): 244–75.

Chapter 9

1. A. Khan et al., "Cinnamon improves glucose and lipids of people with type 2 diabetes." *Diabetes Care* 26, no. 12 (December 2003): 3215–18.
2. J. H. Suh et al.,"Decline in transcriptional activity of Nrf2 causes age-related loss of glutathione synthesis, which is reversible with lipoic acid." *Proceedings of the National Academy of Sciences* 101, no. 10 (March 2004): 3381-86.
3. P. Carter, L. Gray, J. Troughton, K. Khunti, M. Davies, "Fruit and vegetable intake and incidence of type 2 diabetes mellitus: a systemic review and meta-analysis," *BMJ* (August 2010) 341: c4229.

Chapter 11

1. K. E. Foster-Schubert, C. M. Alfano, and C. R. Duggan, "Effect of diet and exercise, alone or combined, on weight and body composition in overweight-to-obese postmenopausal women." *Obesity* 20, no. 8 (August 2012): 1628–38. Epub 2011 April 14.
2. J. W. Bea et al., "Resistance training predicts 6-yr body composition change in postmenopausal women." *Medicine and Science in Sports and Exercise* 42, no. 7 (July 2010): 1286–95.
3. Jan-Willem van Dijk, K. Tummers, and C. D. A. Stehouwer, "Exercise therapy in type 2 diabetes: Is daily exercise required to optimize glycemic control?" *Diabetes Care* 35, no. 5 (May 2012): 948–54. Epub 2012 March 7.
4. N. Brooks et al., "Strength training improves muscle quality and insulin sensitivity in Hispanic older adults with type 2 diabetes." *International Journal of Medical Sciences* 4, no. 1 (18 December 2006): 19–27.
5. K. J. Stewart et al.,"Exercise effects on cardiac size and left ventricular diastolic function: Relationships to changes in fitness, fatness, blood pressure and insulin resistance." *Heart* 92, no. 7 (July 2006) 893–98. Epub 2005 November 24.
6. A. G. Huebschmann, W. M. Kohrt, and J. G. Regensteiner, "Exercise attenuates the premature cardiovascular aging effects of type 2 diabetes mellitus." *Vascular Medicine* 16, no. 5 (October 2011): 378-90. Epub 2011 September 5.
7. G. Kolata, "Diabetes Study Ends Early with a Surprising Result." *New York Times* (19 October 2012).
8. M. Eliakim et al., "Effect of rhythm on the recovery from intense exercise." *The Journal of Strength & Conditioning Research* 27, no. 4 (2013): 1019–1024.

Chapter 12

1. M. L. Klem et al., "A descriptive study of individuals successful at long-term maintenance of substantial weight loss." *American Journal of Clinical Nutrition* 66, no. 2 (August 1997): 239-246.

Index

Reader's Digest

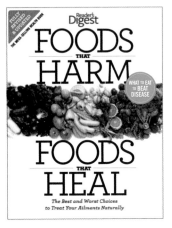

This book changed the way our nation looked at food and its impact on our bodies. This fully revised and updated edition includes hundreds of A-to-Z entries updated with scientific, nutritional, and medical information reflective of the latest research—all in a new reader-friendly format.

$18.99 paperback
Over 500 photos & illustrations

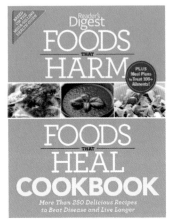

An all-new cookbook companion to the groundbreaking, bestselling health book. Inside you'll find more than 250 scrumptious recipes and sample daily meal plans for almost 100 common ailments, from arthritis to heart disease, as well as an A-to-Z summary of healing foods with buying, storing, and cooking tips.

$19.99 paperback
Full-color photos throughout

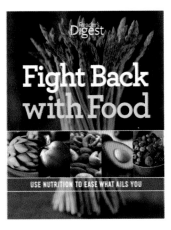

An easy-to-use reference arranged in A-to-Z format, packed with nutrition tips for a healthier life. Part 1 reveals 50 superstar foods with the most potential to treat and prevent disease. Part 2 provides a powerful food arsenal to help fight 50 common ailments. Part 3 has over 100 recipes for treating and fighting disease.

$17.95 paperback
Over 200 photos & illustrations

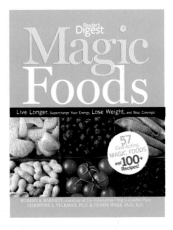

Discover 57 magic foods that can change your life, with 100 appetizing recipes designed to rein in insulin resistance, offload dangerous belly fat, guard against diabetes, and leave you ready to embrace life.

$17.95 paperback
Over 100 photos & illustrations